Regulation of Vascular Smooth Muscle Function

Integrated Systems Physiology: From Molecule to Function

Editors

D. Neil Granger, *Louisiana State University Health Sciences Center*

Joey P. Granger, *University of Mississippi Medical Center*

Physiology is a scientific discipline devoted to understanding the functions of the body. It addresses function at multiple levels, including molecular, cellular, organ, and system. An appreciation of the processes that occur at each level is necessary to understand function in health and the dysfunction associated with disease. Homeostasis and integration are fundamental principles of physiology that account for the relative constancy of organ processes and bodily function even in the face of substantial environmental changes. This constancy results from integrative, cooperative interactions of chemical and electrical signaling processes within and between cells, organs and systems. This eBook series on the broad field of physiology covers the major organ systems from an integrative perspective that addresses the molecular and cellular processes that contribute to homeostasis. Material on pathophysiology is also included throughout the eBooks. The state-of the-art treatises were produced by leading experts in the field of physiology. Each eBook includes stand-alone information and is intended to be of value to students, scientists, and clinicians in the biomedical sciences. Since physiological concepts are an ever-changing work-in-progress, each contributor will have the opportunity to make periodic updates of the covered material.

Published titles

(for future titles please see the website, www.morganclaypool.com/page/lifesci)

Control of Cardiac Output

David B. Young

2010

The Gastrointestinal Circulation

Peter R. Kvietys

2010

Capillary Fluid Exchange: Regulation, Functions, and Pathology
Joshua Scallan, Virgina H. Huxley, and Ronald J. Korthuis
2010

Platelet-Vessel Wall Interactions in Hemostasis and Thrombosis
Rolando Rumbault and Perumal Thiagarajan
2010

The Cerebral Circulation
Marilyn J. Cipolla
2009

Hepatic Circulation
W. Wayne Lautt
2009

Regulation of Vascular Smooth Muscle Function
Raouf A. Khalil
www.morganclaypool.com

ISBN: 9781615041800 paperback

ISBN: 9781615041817 ebook

DOI: 10.4199/C00012ED1V01Y201005ISP007

A Publication in the Morgan & Claypool Publishers series

INTEGRATED SYSTEMS PHYSIOLOGY: FROM MOLECULE TO FUNCTION

Book #7

Series Editors: D. Neil Granger, Louisiana State University Health Sciences Center; Joey P. Granger, University of Mississippi Medical Center

Series ISSN

ISSN 2154-560X   print

ISSN 2154-5626   electronic

Regulation of Vascular Smooth Muscle Function

Raouf A. Khalil
Brigham and Women's Hospital and Harvard Medical School
Boston, Massachusetts

INTEGRATED SYSTEMS PHYSIOLOGY: FROM MOLECULE TO FUNCTION #7

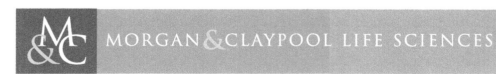

ABSTRACT

Vascular smooth muscle (VSM) constitutes most of the tunica media in blood vessels and plays an important role in the control of vascular tone. Ca^{2+} is a major regulator of VSM contraction and is strictly regulated by an intricate system of Ca^{2+} mobilization and Ca^{2+} homeostatic mechanisms. The interaction of a physiological agonist with its plasma membrane receptor stimulates the hydrolysis of membrane phospholipids and increases the generation of inositol 1,4,5-trisphosphate (IP_3) and diacylglycerol (DAG). IP_3 stimulates Ca^{2+} release from the intracellular stores in the sarcoplasmic reticulum. Agonists also stimulate Ca^{2+} influx from the extracellular space via voltage-gated, receptor-operated, and store-operated channels. Ca^{2+} homeostatic mechanisms tend to decrease the intracellular free Ca^{2+} concentration ($[Ca^{2+}]_i$) by activating Ca^{2+} extrusion via the plasmalemmal Ca^{2+} pump and the Na^+/Ca^{2+} exchanger and the uptake of excess Ca^{2+} by the sarcoplasmic reticulum and possibly the mitochondria. A threshold increase in $[Ca^{2+}]_i$ activates Ca^{2+}-dependent myosin light chain (MLC) phosphorylation, stimulates actin–myosin interaction, and initiates VSM contraction. The agonist-induced maintained increase in DAG also activates specific protein kinase C (PKC) isoforms, which in turn cause phosphorylation of cytoplasmic substrates that increase the contractile myofilaments force sensitivity to Ca^{2+} and thereby enhance VSM contraction. Agonists could also activate Rho kinase (ROCK), leading to inhibition of MLC phosphatase and further enhancement of the myofilaments force sensitivity to Ca^{2+}. The combined increases in $[Ca^{2+}]_i$, PKC and ROCK activity cause significant vasoconstriction and could also stimulate VSM hypertrophy and hyperplasia. The protracted and progressive activation of these processes could lead to pathological vascular remodeling and vascular disease.

KEYWORDS

signal transduction; vascular smooth muscle; calcium; blood pressure; AngII, angiotensin II; ATP, adenosine triphosphate; CPI-17, PKC-potentiated phosphatase inhibitor protein-17 kDa; CAM, calmodulin; DAG, diacylglycerol; ET-1, endothelin; IP_3, inositol 1,4,5-trisphosphate; MAPK, mitogen-activated protein kinase; MARCKs, myristoylated alanine-rich C-kinase substrate; MEK, MAPK kinase; MLC, myosin light chain; NCX, $Na^+–Ca^{2+}$ exchanger; PDBu, phorbol 12,13-dibutyrate; PIP_2, phosphatidylinositol 4,5-bisphosphate; PKC, protein kinase C; PMA, phorbol myristate acetate; RACKs, receptors for activated C-kinase; ROCK, Rho-kinase; VSMC, vascular smooth muscle cell

ix

Acknowledgments

This work was supported by grants from the National Heart, Lung, and Blood Institute (HL-65998) and the Eunice Kennedy Shriver National Institute of Child Health and Human Development (HD-60702).

Contents

CHAPTER 1

Introduction

Vascular smooth muscle (VSM) contraction plays an important role in the regulation of vascular resistance and blood pressure, and its dysregulation may lead to vascular diseases such as hypertension and coronary artery disease. VSM contraction is triggered by an increase in intracellular free Ca^{2+} concentration ($[Ca^{2+}]_i$) due to Ca^{2+} release from the intracellular stores in the smooth sarcoplasmic reticulum and Ca^{2+} entry from the extracellular space through the plasma membrane Ca^{2+} channels [1]. The Ca^{2+} concentration is several-fold higher in the sarcoplasmic reticulum and the extracellular space than in the cytosol. Therefore, the opening of Ca^{2+} channels in the sarcoplasmic reticulum membrane causes Ca^{2+} release into the cytosol. On the other hand, the opening of surface membrane Ca^{2+} channels allows Ca^{2+} to enter from the extracellular space into the cytosol.

Ca^{2+} binds calmodulin (CAM) to form a Ca^{2+}–CAM complex, which activates myosin light chain (MLC) kinase and causes MLC phosphorylation, actin–myosin interaction, and VSM contraction (Figure 1.1). VSM relaxation is initiated by a decrease in $[Ca^{2+}]_i$ due to Ca^{2+} uptake by the sarcoplasmic reticulum Ca^{2+} pump and Ca^{2+} extrusion via the plasmalemmal Ca^{2+} pump and Na^+–Ca^{2+} exchanger. The decrease in $[Ca^{2+}]_i$ causes dissociation of the Ca^{2+}–CAM complex, and the phosphorylated MLC is dephosphorylated by MLC phosphatase [1].

Under physiological conditions, agonist activation of VSM results in an initial phasic contraction followed by a tonic contraction. The initial agonist-induced contraction is generally believed to be due to Ca^{2+} release from the intracellular stores. Although VSM is unique in that it can sustain contraction with minimal energy expense, the mechanisms involved in the maintained VSM contraction are not clearly understood. Ca^{2+}-dependent MLC phosphorylation is a major determinant of the maintained agonist-induced contraction of VSM. However, the classic Ca^{2+}-dependent MLC phosphorylation pathway does not totally explain all modes of maintained VSM contraction and other mechanisms have been suggested. Activation of protein kinase C (PKC) may increase the myofilament force sensitivity to $[Ca^{2+}]_i$ and MLC phosphorylation, and thereby maintain VSM contraction with smaller increases in $[Ca^{2+}]_i$. PKC comprises a family of Ca^{2+}-dependent and Ca^{2+}-independent isoforms, which have different tissue and subcellular distribution and undergo differential translocation during cell activation. PKC translocation to the cell surface may trigger a cascade of protein kinases such as mitogen-activated protein kinase (MAPK) and MAPK kinase

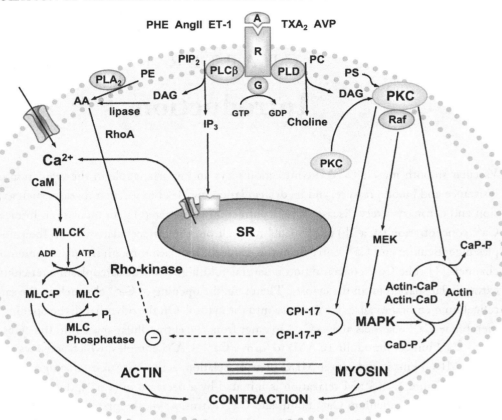

FIGURE 1.1: Mechanisms of VSM contraction. Agonist (A) binds to its receptor (R), stimulates plasma membrane PLCβ, and increases production of IP_3 and diacylglycerol (DAG). IP_3 stimulates Ca^{2+} release from the sarcoplasmic reticulum (SR). Agonist also stimulates Ca^{2+} influx through Ca^{2+} channels. Ca^{2+} binds calmodulin (CAM), activates MLC kinase (MLCK), causes MLC phosphorylation, and initiates VSM contraction. DAG activates PKC. PKC phosphorylates CPI-17, which in turn inhibits MLC phosphatase and thereby enhances the myofilament force sensitivity to Ca^{2+}. PKC could phosphorylate calponin (Cap), allowing more actin to bind myosin. PKC may activate a protein kinase cascade involving Raf, MAPK kinase (MEK), and MAPK, leading to phosphorylation of the actin-binding protein caldesmon (CaD). Other pathways of VSM contraction include the RhoA/Rho-kinase pathway, which inhibits MLC phosphatase and further enhances the Ca^{2+} sensitivity. G, heterotrimeric G-protein; PIP_2, phosphatidylinositol 4,5-bisphosphate; PC, phosphatidylcholine; PS, phosphatidylserine; PE, phosphatidylethanolamine; AA, arachidonic acid.

(MEK) that ultimately interact with the contractile myofilaments and cause VSM contraction. Additional signaling pathways such as Rho-kinase could further enhance the myofilament force sensitivity to $[Ca^{2+}]_i$. These Ca^{2+}-dependent and Ca^{2+}-sensitization pathways work synergistically during the development and maintenance of agonist-induced contraction of VSM [2–4]. The role of Ca^{2+} and other signaling pathways of VSM contraction will be discussed.

CHAPTER 2

Ca^{2+} Release from the Intracellular Stores

Stimulation of VSM by various physiological agonists produces a transient contractile response in the absence of extracellular Ca^{2+} [1,5]. Also, while pretreatment of vascular segments with Ca^{2+} channel blockers significantly inhibits ^{45}Ca^{2+} influx and the maintained agonist-induced contraction, a smaller transient contraction can still be elicited under these conditions [1,5,6]. In addition, agonists stimulate Ca^{2+} efflux from ^{45}Ca^{2+} loaded vascular segments, particularly in a Ca^{2+}-free medium [7]. These observations have suggested that Ca^{2+} release from an intracellular Ca^{2+} storage site may contribute to the agonist-induced VSM contraction [1].

Ultrastructure studies in smooth muscle have revealed structures consistent with the sarcoplasmic reticulum, and electron probe X-ray microanalysis has shown that this organelle can accumulate Ca^{2+} from solutions containing micromolar concentrations of Ca^{2+} [8]. The sarcoplasmic reticulum is an intracellular membrane system of tubules and, in some species, flattened cisternae [8,9]. It occupies from 1.5% to 7.5% of the smooth muscle cell volume [10]. The largest volume of the sarcoplasmic reticulum is encountered in large elastic arteries, such as the rabbit main pulmonary artery, a blood vessel that also elicits a large contraction in the absence of extracellular Ca^{2+}. In contrast, phasic smooth muscle such as the guinea pig taenia coli and the rabbit mesenteric vein contain relatively small volume (1.5–2.5%) of sarcoplasmic reticulum and therefore lose their responsiveness more readily in Ca^{2+}-free solution. However, even this small volume of sarcoplasmic reticulum can store sufficient Ca^{2+} for activating a near maximal contraction when released [11].

The sarcoplasmic reticulum has been isolated as a microsomal fraction using advanced biochemical techniques. Isolated smooth muscle microsomes have been shown to accumulate ^{45}Ca^{2+} and to release it in response to Ca^{2+}-releasing agents such as caffeine. Also, the Ca^{2+} release channel in sarcoplasmic reticulum vesicles of smooth muscle has been characterized in planar lipid bilayer [12]. Importantly, chemical skinning of smooth muscle preparations using saponin or α-toxin has circumvented the loss of some of the essential cellular components during isolation and purification of the sarcoplasmic reticulum vesicles and thereby enabled investigators to study the Ca^{2+} release mechanism under more physiological conditions [9,13–16]. Ca^{2+} release from the sarcoplasmic reticulum is triggered by two intracellular second messengers, namely, inositol 1,4,5-trisphosphate (IP_3) and Ca^{2+}.

2.1   INOSITOL TRISPHOSPHATE-INDUCED Ca^{2+} RELEASE

One of the earliest biochemical events that follows the agonist–receptor interaction is stimulation of the membrane-associated phospholipase C, which stimulates the breakdown of the plasma membrane phosphatidylinositol 4,5-bisphosphate (PIP_2) into 1,2-diacylglycerol (DAG) and IP_3 [17]. DAG is a lipophilic compound that remains in the plasma membrane where it binds to and activates PKC [3,18]. On the other hand, IP_3 is a water-soluble compound that diffuses in the cytosol and

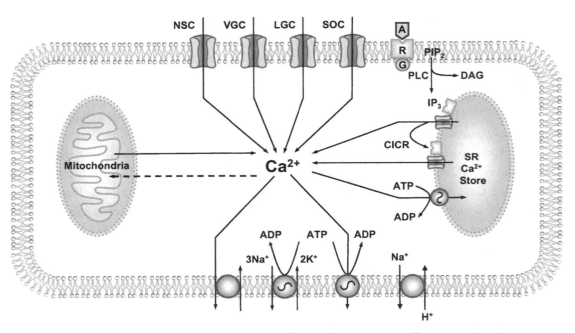

FIGURE 2.1: Schematic representation of the Ca^{2+} mobilization and Ca^{2+} homeostatic mechanisms in vascular smooth muscle. Intracellular Ca^{2+} stores in the sarcoplasmic reticulum (SR) are released in response to 1,4,5-inositol trisphosphate (IP_3) or to Ca^{2+} via Ca^{2+}-induced Ca^{2+} release (CICR). Extracellular Ca^{2+} enters the cell through the passive Ca^{2+} leak or nonspecific Ca^{2+} channels (NSC), receptor-operated or ligand-gated Ca^{2+} channels (LGC), voltage-gated Ca^{2+} channels (VGC), and store-operated channels (SOC). The increased intracellular Ca^{2+} is taken up by the sarcoplasmic reticulum Ca^{2+} pump or extruded by the plasmalemmal Ca^{2+} pump. At high intracellular Ca^{2+} concentrations, the Na^+–Ca^{2+} exchanger and the mitochondria may play a role in Ca^{2+} homeostasis. A. agonist; R. receptor; G, guanosine triphosphate-binding protein; PIP_2, phosphatidylinositol 4,5-bisphosphate; PLC, phospholipase C.

stimulates Ca^{2+} release from the sarcoplasmic reticulum [19-22] (Figure 2.1). Studies in smooth muscle cells chemically skinned with saponin have shown that the IP_3-induced Ca^{2+} release is large and rapid. The half maximal effective concentration of IP_3 (~1 μM) is low enough to account for the observed transient smooth muscle contraction [19,21,23]. Also, a specific phosphatase, which rapidly inactivates IP_3, in accordance with the requirements for its function as a second messenger has been identified in smooth muscle [24]. IP_3 binds to a specific receptor on the surface of the sarcoplasmic reticulum where it activates an IP_3-sensitive Ca^{2+} release channel. Heparin, likely via its electronegative charge, competes with IP_3 for its receptor and thus inhibits IP_3-induced Ca^{2+} release from the sarcoplasmic reticulum [25].

2.2   Ca²⁺-INDUCED Ca²⁺ RELEASE

Small concentrations of Ca^{2+} have been shown to induce further Ca^{2+} release from the sarcoplasmic reticulum of skinned skeletal [9,26]), cardiac muscle [27], and VSM [13]. Ca^{2+}-induced Ca^{2+} release (CICR) is a regenerative process that can be facilitated by Ca^{2+}-releasing agents such as caffeine [9]. CICR is triggered when the concentration of Ca^{2+} near the sarcoplasmic reticulum exceeds a threshold of 3×10^{-6} M. The threshold Ca^{2+} concentration that stimulates Ca^{2+} release is increased in the presence of Mg^{2+}. CICR is enhanced by adenosine $3',5'$-cyclic monophosphate (cyclic AMP) and inhibited by procaine [13].

In contrast to skeletal and cardiac muscle, an influx of extracellular Ca^{2+} is not necessary to stimulate CICR from smooth muscle sarcoplasmic reticulum. However, an increase in Ca^{2+} concentration in the vicinity of the sarcoplasmic reticulum is essential for this regenerative process to take place. It has been suggested that an initial IP_3-induced Ca^{2+} release from the sarcoplasmic reticulum through a subset of Ca^{2+} release channels could raise Ca^{2+} concentration near the sarcoplasmic reticulum above the threshold of 3×10^{-6} M, which in turn stimulates more Ca^{2+} release from the sarcoplasmic reticulum through a second subset of Ca^{2+} release channels [28]. This signaling amplification system is supported by the observation that Ca^{2+} enhances IP_3-induced Ca^{2+} release from the sarcoplasmic reticulum in skinned smooth muscle preparations [23].

·　·　·　·　·

CHAPTER 3

Ca^{2+} Entry from the Extracellular Space

Several Ca^{2+} entry pathways have been identified or suggested in VSM cells (VSMCs) including the Ca^{2+} leak, voltage-gated Ca^{2+} channels, receptor-operated Ca^{2+} channels (ROCCs), store-operated Ca^{2+} channels (SOCCs), and stretch-activated Ca^{2+} channels (Figure 2.1).

3.1   Ca^{2+} LEAK

Ca^{2+} leak is defined as the Ca^{2+} entry pathway through which Ca^{2+} passes down its electrochemical gradient into the resting cell. This Ca^{2+} entry pathway is probably lined with both phosphate and carboxyl groups because it is partially blocked by increasing the hydrogen ion concentration. Also, inorganic trivalent cations such as lanthanum and divalent cations such as cobalt have been shown to block the Ca^{2+} leak by ~66% [1].

It has generally been thought that the Ca^{2+} leak represents Ca^{2+} movements that do not require the opening of specific Ca^{2+} channels. However, Benham and Tsien [29] have described a divalent cation-selective channel that displays occasional spontaneous openings and may contribute to the Ca^{2+} leak. This channel opens at holding potentials below the threshold for activation of voltage-gated Ca^{2+} channel and has a higher conductance than the adenosine triphosphate (ATP)-sensitive Ca^{2+} channel (an ROCC), and therefore has been designated as a separate type of channel.

The magnitude of the Ca^{2+} leak in VSMCs has been determined by ^{45}Ca^{2+} flux measurements. In rabbit aorta at rest, ^{45}Ca^{2+} influx is ~14 µmol/kg/min [5]. This large Ca^{2+} leak does not cause VSM contraction because it is constantly balanced by Ca^{2+} homeostatic mechanisms such as Ca^{2+} uptake by the sarcoplasmic reticulum and Ca^{2+} extrusion to the extracellular space. If these Ca^{2+} homeostatic mechanisms are compromised or the myofilament force sensitivity to Ca^{2+} is increased, the Ca^{2+} leak pathway could contribute to VSM contraction.

3.2   VOLTAGE-GATED Ca^{2+} CHANNELS

The presence of extracellular Ca^{2+} is essential for maintained contraction of certain types of VSM in response to certain stimuli [1]. In rabbit aorta, force development in response to membrane depolarization by high K$^+$ solution is abolished in the absence of extracellular Ca^{2+}. Also, the maintained norepinephrine-induced contraction in rabbit aorta is significantly inhibited in Ca^{2+}-free medium. The magnitude of Ca^{2+} entry into VSM cell during activation by various agonists has been determined by measuring $^{45}Ca^{2+}$ influx using radioactive isotopes [30] and Ca^{2+} current using electrophysiology and patch-clamp techniques [31–34]. Measurement of Ca^{2+} influx has shown that the Ca^{2+} entry induced by high K^+ depolarizing solution is sensitive to organic Ca^{2+} antagonists, particularly the dihydropyridines group [6]. Also, a strong correlation has been found between the Ca^{2+} antagonist-induced blockade of $^{45}Ca^{2+}$ influx and parallel inhibition of vascular contraction [1]. Furthermore, Bay K8644, a Ca^{2+} channel agonist, has been shown to stimulate Ca^{2+} influx and to induce vascular contraction, thus establishing a causal link between both parameters. These observations have suggested a distinct Ca^{2+} entry pathway in the plasma membrane that is activated by membrane depolarization and has been termed *voltage-gated Ca^{2+} channels (VGCCs)* [35–37].

The advent of the voltage-clamp and patch-clamp techniques has provided further characterization of the VGCCs in VSMCs. Most of these studies have provided evidence for two components of voltage-activated Ca^{2+} current, one of which is activated by relatively large depolarizations and inactivates relatively slowly, while the other is activated by relatively small depolarizations and inactivates relatively rapidly. These two components have been referred to as L and T currents, respectively [33]. Both components of the Ca^{2+} current are blocked by lanthanum [31], cadmium [34,38], and cobalt [32,34], but can be distinguished by their sensitivity to dihydropyridines. The L current is blocked by dihydropyridines such as nisoldipine, nimodipine, nifedipine, and nitrendipine and is augmented by Bay K8644 and Bay R5417. In contrast, the T current is not significantly affected by these dihydropyridines [31–34].

An important question is whether VGCCs are modulated by physiological agonists. Some studies have shown that norepinephrine has no effect on the voltage-activated Ca^{2+} current [31–34]. However, in the rabbit ear artery, norepinephrine, acting via a non-α non-β receptor, stimulates the L-type current but not the T-type current [39]. Also, in rabbit mesenteric artery, norepinephrine can activate and increase the open probability of VGCCs [37].

3.3 RECEPTOR-OPERATED (LIGAND-GATED) Ca²⁺ CHANNELS

While the high K^+-induced VSM contraction and Ca^{2+} influx are sensitive to Ca^{2+} channel antagonists, the VSM contraction and Ca^{2+} influx induced by physiological agonists such as norepinephrine are refractory to organic Ca^{2+} antagonists. On the other hand, these agonists still require extracellular Ca^{2+} to produce maximal and maintained vascular contraction. In rabbit aorta, norepinephrine causes further increase in contraction after maximal depolarization of the tissue by high K^+ solution. Also, $^{45}Ca^{2+}$ influx stimulated by simultaneous application of maximal concentrations of norepinephrine and high K^+ depolarizing solution is equal to the sum of that stimulated by each one alone, that is, the norepinephrine and high K^+-induced Ca^{2+} influx are additive. Furthermore, the $^{45}Ca^{2+}$ influx stimulated by Ca^{2+} channel agonists such as Bay K8644 is additive to that induced by maximal concentrations of norepinephrine but not to that induced by high K$^+$ [1,40]. These ob-servations have suggested that physiological agonists activate Ca^{2+} channels that are different from those activated by membrane depolarization and have been termed *receptor-operated Ca^{2+} channels* or *ligand-gated Ca^{2+} channels* [35,36].

Electrophysiological studies have provided more direct evidence for ROCCs. Benham and Tsien [29] have reported that ATP activates a distinct Ca^{2+} current in the rabbit ear artery. The ATP-sensitive channel displays a 3:1 selectivity for Ca^{2+} over Na$^+$ at near physiological ionic con-ditions. It can be distinguished from the VGCC by its insensitivity to blockade by nifedipine and cadmium, its opening at high negative potentials, and its unitary conductance of ~5 pS in 110 mM Ca^{2+} or Ba^{2+}. Since the channel is not activated when ATP is added outside the cell-attached patch pipette, it appears to be directly coupled to receptor activation by ATP rather than through an ATP-induced generation of a freely diffusible messenger [41].

3.4   STORE-OPERATED Ca^{2+} CHANNELS

As described above, the release of intracellular Ca^{2+} occurs from the sarcoplasmic reticulum in response to second messengers such as IP$_3$. The release of Ca^{2+} from intracellular stores is often followed by sustained Ca^{2+} entry from the extracellular space [42–44]. This led to the suggestion that depleted Ca^{2+} stores in the endoplasmic reticulum act as a capacitor for stimulated maintained Ca^{2+} entry from the extracellular space and has been defined as "capacitative Ca^{2+} entry" and later as "store-operated Ca^{2+} entry" [43–45]. This was later supported by the identification of store-operated Ca^{2+} release-activated Ca^{2+} current [46,47].

The functional significance of store-operated Ca^{2+} entry has been examined using selec-tive inhibitors of the sarcoplasmic/endoplasmic reticulum Ca^{2+}-ATPase (SERCA) such as cyclo-piazonic acid and thapsigargin. These compounds cause depletion of sarcoplasmic reticulum Ca^{2+} stores by inhibiting sequestration of Ca^{2+} ions without activation of guanosine triphosphate (GTP)-binding proteins and thereby differentiate between Ca^{2+} entering through SOCCs and ROCCs. In effect, sustained Ca^{2+} influx or cellular responses during treatment by sarcoplasmic reticulum Ca^{2+}-ATPase inhibitors is often used as markers for the involvement of SOCC in cell signaling. In cultured VSMCs, depletion of sarcoplasmic reticulum Ca^{2+} stores with thapsigargin activates Ca^{2+} influx that is independent of the generation of inositol phosphate and resistant to the L-type VGCC blocker nicardipine [48]. SERCA inhibitors not only increase Ca^{2+} influx but also maintain vascular tone that is dependent on extracellular Ca^{2+} [49,50].

The cellular mechanisms by which SOCCs are activated have not been clearly established. Studies in mouse aortic VSM cells suggested that the depletion of Ca^{2+} stores triggers the re-lease of a Ca^{2+} influx factor (CIF), which activates SOCCs [51]. Other studies have identified a 3-pS Ca^{2+}-conducting channel that is activated by 1,2-bis(*o*-aminophenoxy)ethane-*N,N,N',N'*-

tetraacetic acid (BAPTA) and thapsigargin and causes passive depletion of intracellular Ca^{2+} stores. The 3-pS channel is also activated in inside-out membrane patches from smooth muscle cells when stimulated by CIF extracted from mutant yeast cell line, making it a likely native SOCC in VSMCs [52]. Although CIF has been partly purified in a stable form, its molecular structure has yet to be defined [53].

Members of the canonical transient receptor potential channels (TRPCs), such as TRPC1, may play a role in store-operated Ca^{2+} entry in VSM [54–56]. TRPC1 may be linked to TRPP2 (polycystin-2) Ca^{2+} permeable channel [57]. TRPC5 may represent another component of SOCCs [58]. Other members of the TRPC family, including TRPC3, TRPC4, and TRPC7, have been associated with store-operated Ca^{2+} entry in nonvascular cells [59,60].

Recent studies have suggested that a membrane-spanning protein termed stromal-interacting molecule 1 (STIM1) may play a role in the activation of SOCCs. STIM1 may serve as a sensor of Ca^{2+} within the stores and may interact with TRPC1 and promote store-operated Ca^{2+} entry [61,62]. Other studies have suggested that Orai1 is a pore subunit of SOCCs [63]. Studies have shown an interaction between STIM1 and Orai1 that could lead to a gain in SOCC function [64,65].

3.5   STRETCH-ACTIVATED Ca^{2+} CHANNELS

During the process of "autoregulation" of peripheral blood flow, an elevation of intravascular pressure and stretch of the vascular wall can produce a maintained increase in VSM tone [66]. Stretch-stimulated vascular tone is highly dependent on extracellular Ca^{2+}, suggesting the activation of a stretch-dependent Ca^{2+} channel [67]. Stretch-activated Ca^{2+} channels differ from VGCCs and ROCCs in their sensitivity to Ca^{2+} antagonists, being more sensitive to diltiazem but insensitive to dihydropyridines. Mechanical stretch stimulates $^{45}Ca^{2+}$ influx and opens nonspecific cation channels in smooth muscle membranes [68]. The mechanism of activation of stretch-sensitive Ca^{2+} channels is not clear, but a role of the endothelium in VSM response to stretch has been suggested [69].

·   ·   ·   ·

CHAPTER 4

Mechanisms of Ca^{2+} Homeostasis

In addition to their role in Ca^{2+} mobilization, the smooth muscle plasma membrane and intracellular organelles also play a role in maintaining cellular Ca^{2+} homeostasis. The plasmalemmal Ca^{2+}-adenosine triphosphatase (Ca^{2+}-ATPase) plays a predominant role in maintaining [Ca^{2+}]$_i$ close to the basal levels, and the Na$^+$–Ca^{2+} exchanger contributes to the removal of excess cytosolic Ca^{2+} (Figure 2.1). In addition to the events occurring at the plasma membrane level, two intracellular organelles determine the cytosolic Ca^{2+} concentration, namely, the sarcoplasmic reticulum and the mitochondria. These organelles have pump-leak system that involves active uptake of Ca^{2+} from the cytosol and passive leak of Ca^{2+} back to the cytosol.

4.1   PLASMALEMMAL Ca^{2+}-ATPASE

Studies have shown that metabolic inhibition of the smooth muscle of guinea pig taenia coli using iodoacetic acid or 2,4-dinitrophenol causes a net Ca^{2+} uptake that is similar in magnitude to the passive Ca^{2+} leak [70,71]. These observations have suggested that an ATP-dependent Ca^{2+} extrusion pump contributes to smooth muscle Ca^{2+} homeostasis and that inhibition of the Ca^{2+} pump causes accumulation of Ca^{2+} inside the cell [72]. The smooth muscle plasmalemmal Ca^{2+} pump is probably similar to the better studied Ca^{2+} pump in the squid axon and red blood cells [73]. The Ca^{2+} pump has a molecular weight of 130 kDa. It is stimulated by calmodulin and inhibited by vanadate. The observation that vanadate causes maximal contraction of VSM suggests that the plasmalemmal Ca^{2+} pump plays a major role in the regulation of [Ca^{2+}]$_i$ and vascular tone [74]. Also, certain agonists such as oxytocin and prostaglandins have been shown to promote smooth muscle contraction in part by inhibiting the plasmalemmal Ca^{2+} extrusion pump [75,76].

The plasmalemmal Ca^{2+}-ATPase can be distinguished from other ATPases in the plasmalemma and endoplasmic reticulum by its insensitivity to ouabain (distinction from Na$^+$,K$^+$-ATPase), high sensitivity to inhibition by vanadate (more sensitive than endoplasmic reticulum ATPase), sensitivity to K$^+$ (less sensitive than endoplasmic reticulum ATPase), and sensitivity to calmodulin antagonists [77].

Molecular biology studies have been successful in molecular cloning and in the purification and amino acid sequencing of the plasmalemmal Ca^{2+} pump from several cell types including smooth muscle [78-80].

4.2   THE SODIUM–CALCIUM EXCHANGER

The Na^+–Ca^{2+} exchanger (NCX) provides an alternative plasma membrane mechanism through which excess intracellular Ca^{2+} is removed to the extracellular space against a large $[Ca^{2+}]$ gradient. The contribution of NCX to Ca^{2+} homeostasis has been suggested in many cell types including smooth muscle [81,82]. Studies on membrane vesicles have shown that an NCX activity copurifies with plasma membrane markers, suggesting a plasmalemmal activity. Also, several research groups have been successful in the isolation and functional reconstitution of the plasmalemmal NCX [83,84]. The plasmalemmal NCX has been distinguished from the mitochondrial NCX by its markedly different specificity and stoichiometry [85].

Some of the questions regarding the exact nature of the plasmalemmal NCX as well as its stoichiometry, direction, and pathophysiological significance have been addressed. NCX is driven by the transmembrane Na^+ and Ca^{2+} gradients and the membrane potential. The energy derived from either Na^+ or Ca^{2+}, moving down its electrochemical gradient, is balanced by an antiport movement of the coupled ion. This transport mechanism is electrogenic [86] and has a stoichiometry of $3Na^+$:Ca^{2+} [87]. In VSM, NCX may play a role in Ca^{2+} extrusion, but its contribution is not well defined and appears to vary in different tissues [88,89].

Although NCX is often thought of as a Ca^{2+} extrusion pathway, it appears that depending on the membrane potential, the transmembrane ionic gradients of Na^+ and Ca^{2+}, and the relative importance of intracellular Ca^{2+}, NCX could contribute to either Ca^{2+} extrusion or Ca^{2+} influx (reverse-mode NCX). The significance of NCX as a source of intracellular Ca^{2+} may be increased in vascular diseases such as hypertension [90].

4.3   SARCOPLASMIC RETICULUM Ca^{2+}-ATPASE

The role of the sarcoplasmic reticulum (SR) Ca^{2+}-ATPase in Ca^{2+} homeostasis has long been recognized in skeletal and cardiac muscles [91]. It has a molecular weight of 100 kDa, a 2:1 stoichiometry between Ca^{2+} transport and ATP hydrolysis, and is phosphorylated by various protein kinases. The ability of SR to accumulate Ca^{2+} is significantly less in other systems including smooth muscle [92]. However, smooth muscle SR microsomes show energy-dependent Ca^{2+} uptake. Also, Ca^{2+} electron probe X-ray microanalysis of saponin-permeabilized smooth muscle has demonstrated a nonmitochondrial ATP-dependent Ca^{2+}-pump activity that is blocked by vanadate [8]. The affinity of the SR pump for Ca^{2+} ($K_m = 0.2$–0.6 μM) is sufficiently high to take up Ca^{2+} and to cause muscle relaxation. Also, a high-capacity low-affinity Ca^{2+}-binding protein known as calsequestrin has been identified in isolated skeletal and smooth muscle SR preparations, and has been shown to increase the SR Ca^{2+} storage capacity [93,94]. However, the capacity of the SR to accumulate Ca^{2+} is limited, and therefore during repeated and excessive Ca^{2+} loads, the mitochondria may become the major Ca^{2+} pool [95].

4.4   MITOCHONDRIA AND Ca^{2+}

Although mitochondria occupy approximately 5% of the total smooth muscle cell volume [8], their role in the regulation of intracellular Ca^{2+} under physiological and pathological conditions has not been fully examined. Also, the concentration of free Ca^{2+} in the mitochondrial matrix space is unclear. There are separate Ca^{2+} influx and Ca^{2+} efflux pathways across the mitochondrial membrane [85,96]. The Ca^{2+} influx pathway operates as a Ca^{2+} uniporter driven by the large mitochondrial membrane potential (150 mV, inside negative), and the Ca^{2+} efflux pathway involves a $Ca^{2+}:2H^+$ or $Ca^{2+}:2Na^+$ antiporter [97,98]. The Ca^{2+} efflux pathway has lower capacity than the Ca^{2+} influx pathway [96]. Under physiological conditions, the major cellular cytosolic anion is phosphate. When Ca^{2+} is taken up by mitochondria, HPO_4^{2-} is also taken up via $HPO_4^{2-}:2OH^-$ exchange and calcium phosphate is formed. According to Mitchell's hypothesis of mitochondrial energy transfer [99], the primary event is the development of an electrochemical proton gradient across the mitochondrial membrane with the pH gradient in mitochondria greater than cytoplasm. In an alkaline environment, the solubility of calcium phosphates is extremely low. Thus, the major determinants of the free $[Ca^{2+}]$ within the mitochondrial matrix space are the extra- and intramitochondrial phosphate concentration, the intramitochondrial pH, and the K_m and V_{max} of the efflux pathway [97]. The role of mitochondria in cellular Ca^{2+} homeostasis can be easily understood by considering the rate of Ca^{2+} uptake into mitochondria as a function of the cytosolic Ca^{2+} concentration. The rate of mitochondrial Ca^{2+} uptake increases dramatically as the cytosolic Ca^{2+} rises to abnormally high levels. Since the Ca^{2+} efflux pathway out of the mitochondria is saturable [96], the rate of mitochondrial Ca^{2+} uptake will exceed the Ca^{2+} efflux rate and a net accumulation of Ca^{2+} by the mitochondria occurs [97]. The accumulated Ca^{2+} then deposits into a nonionic calcium pool of calcium phosphate. Thus, the mitochondria function as a sink for Ca^{2+} during Ca^{2+} overload. The mitochondrial free Ca^{2+}, however, is in equilibrium with the large nonionic calcium pool. This arrangement means that the cytosolic free Ca^{2+} is coupled to the nonionic calcium pool in the mitochondria. Consequently, when the cytosolic free Ca^{2+} is lower than the mitochondrial free Ca^{2+}, the nonionic calcium pool is released to stabilize the cytosolic free Ca^{2+}. On the other hand, when the cytosolic Ca^{2+} is within the normal basal level (~0.1 μM), the mitochondrial free Ca^{2+} will have a similar value and the plasma membrane and the SR will be largely responsible for maintaining the cellular Ca^{2+} homeostasis. Also, because the capacity of the mitochondria, although large, is finite, it is presumed that they slowly release their stored calcium during periods of cellular quiescence when it can be handled by the plasmalemmal and SR Ca^{2+} pumps. Thus, the SR may play the major physiological role as the Ca^{2+} storage site, and the mitochondria accumulate Ca^{2+} only when cytosolic Ca^{2+} is abnormally high, exceeding 5 μM [8,100]. The apparent K_m of mitochondria for Ca^{2+} uptake is approximately 10–17 μM, which is higher than that of the SR (K_m ~1 μM). Therefore, smooth muscle mitochondria are minimally loaded with Ca^{2+} under physiological conditions [8,100]. Thus, the mitochondrial large Ca^{2+} buffering capacity plays a role in the regulation of cytoplasmic Ca^{2+} only under pathological conditions when "Ca^{2+} overload" occurs, that is, when cell viability is threatened by massive Ca^{2+} influx. The high Ca^{2+} content of mitochondria isolated from atherosclerotic blood vessels may reflect smooth muscle damage, and such cells containing calcium-loaded mitochondria may become the initial sites of vascular calcification [8].

·　·　·　·　·

CHAPTER 5

Ca^{2+}-Dependent Myosin Light Chain Phosphorylation

5.1 INTRACELLULAR FREE Ca^{2+} CONCENTRATION

$[Ca^{2+}]_i$ is regulated by a balance between the Ca^{2+} mobilizing mechanisms that increase $[Ca^{2+}]_i$ (i.e., Ca^{2+} release from the sarcoplasmic reticulum and Ca^{2+} influx from the extracellular space) and the Ca^{2+} homeostatic mechanisms that decrease $[Ca^{2+}]_i$ (i.e., the plasmalemmal and sarcoplasmic reticulum Ca^{2+}-ATPases, the Na$^+$–Ca^{2+} exchanger, and the mitochondria).

$[Ca^{2+}]_i$ has been measured by loading the cells with Ca^{2+} indicators. $[Ca^{2+}]_i$ was first measured in large cells that permit microinjection of suitable metallochromic dyes such as arsenazo III and antipyralzo III [101] or bioluminescent proteins such as aequorin [102,103], or impalement of the cell with Ca^{2+}-sensitive microelectrodes [104]. However, small-sized cells such as smooth muscle may not be suitable for microinjection and impalement techniques. This problem was first circumvented by loading VSM with aequorin using a transient cell permeabilization method [105]. Thereafter, several fluorescent Ca^{2+} indicators have been developed for measuring $[Ca^{2+}]_i$ in many cell types including smooth muscle [106,107]. Fluorescent Ca^{2+} indicators are available in both the free acid Ca^{2+}-sensitive form and the acetoxymethyl ester form. The nonpolar acetoxymethyl ester is more lipophilic and diffuses across the plasma membrane into the cell where it is hydrolyzed by intracellular esterases into the free acid form, acetic acid, and methyl alcohol. The Ca^{2+} indicator free acid form, being more hydrophilic, does not cross the plasma membrane and therefore accumulates inside the cell. This group of fluorescent Ca^{2+} indicators includes quin-2, fura-2, and indo-1 [106–110]. Regardless of the technique used, there is a general agreement among most methods that the physiological $[Ca^{2+}]_i$ is in the range between 0.1 and 1 μM.

5.2 Ca^{2+}-DEPENDENT MYOSIN LIGHT CHAIN PHOSPHORYLATION

It is widely accepted that a major determinant of smooth muscle contraction is the reversible Ca^{2+}-dependent phosphorylation of the 20-kDa MLC [111,112]. Agonist-induced activation of plasma membrane receptors causes an increase in $[Ca^{2+}]_i$ due to initial Ca^{2+} release from the sarcoplasmic reticulum and maintained Ca^{2+} entry from the extracellular space [1]. According to the thick-filament regulation hypothesis of smooth muscle contraction, Ca^{2+} binds CAM to form a Ca^{2+}–CAM complex, which activates MLC kinase (MLCK). Activation of MLCK results in the phosphorylation of the 20-kDa MLC [111,112]. The phosphorylated MLC increases the activity of actin-activated Mg^{2+}-ATPase leading to actin–myosin interaction and smooth muscle contraction (see Figure 1.1). Smooth muscle relaxation is initiated by a decrease in $[Ca^{2+}]_i$ due to Ca^{2+} uptake by the sarcoplasmic reticulum and Ca^{2+} extrusion by the plasmalemmal Ca^{2+} pump and the Na^+–Ca^{2+} exchanger. The decrease in $[Ca^{2+}]_i$ causes dissociation of the Ca^{2+}–CAM complex and the phosphorylated MLC is dephosphorylated by MLC phosphatase.

5.3   EVIDENCE FOR OTHER MECHANISMS OF SMOOTH MUSCLE CONTRACTION

Data from several laboratories have suggested that agonist-induced vascular tone cannot be explained only by Ca^{2+}-dependent MLC phosphorylation. For example, in rabbit aortic rings incubated in Ca^{2+}-free (2 mM EGTA) solution, the α-adrenergic agonist phenylephrine causes a transient increase in contraction followed by a smaller but maintained contraction [5]. The initial increase in contraction can be explained by Ca^{2+} release from the intracellular stores. Also, the large decline in contraction can be explained by the absence of Ca^{2+} influx in the Ca^{2+}-free solution. However, the remaining significant phenylephrine contraction in Ca^{2+}-free solution cannot be easily explained by Ca^{2+}-dependent MLC phosphorylation, suggesting that phenylephrine may activate other mechanisms that increase the myofilament force sensitivity to Ca^{2+}.

Simultaneous measurement of force and $[Ca^{2+}]_i$ in various VSM preparations has been used to determine the effect of agonists on the myofilament force sensitivity to Ca^{2+} [105,113]. In rabbit inferior vena cava loaded with the Ca^{2+} indicator fura-2, norepinephrine causes a rapid initial contraction followed by a maintained contraction. The norepinephrine contraction is accompanied by a rapid $[Ca^{2+}]_i$ spike followed by a smaller but sustained increase in $[Ca^{2+}]_i$ above basal levels. In contrast, membrane depolarization by high K^+ solution causes a maintained increase in contraction and $[Ca^{2+}]_i$. Also, in the rabbit inferior vena cava, for approximately the same steady-state increase in $[Ca^{2+}]_i$, norepinephrine causes greater contraction than that induced by high K^+. The relationship between steady-state $[Ca^{2+}]_i$ and force has also been constructed by maximally stimulating fura-2 loaded inferior vena with norepinephrine or high K^+ in Ca^{2+}-free solution, then increasing concentrations of extracellular Ca^{2+} are added and the simultaneous changes in force and $[Ca^{2+}]_i$ are recorded. These studies have shown that the norepinephrine $[Ca^{2+}]_i$–force relationship is enhanced and located to the left of that induced by high K^+ suggesting that norepinephrine increases the myofilament force sensitivity to Ca^{2+} in rabbit inferior vena cava [113].

Agonist-induced dissociations between $[Ca^{2+}]_i$ and force have been reported in other smooth muscle preparations such as ferret aorta [114], swine carotid artery [115], and rabbit pulmonary artery [116]. Also, agonist-induced dissociations between $[Ca^{2+}]_i$ and MLC phosphorylation have been reported and have been explained by agonist-induced G protein-mediated change in the MLCK/MLC phosphatase activity ratio [117]. However, agonist-induced dissociations between MLC phosphorylation and force have also been demonstrated [118,119]. These agonist-induced dissociations between MLC phosphorylation and force have initially been explained by the "latch bridge" hypothesis, which proposes that the dephosphorylation of myosin may generate a slowly cycling cross-bridge that supports force maintenance [120]. However, the agonist-induced dissociations between MLC phosphorylation and force have not been fully explained by the "latch" hypothesis. That led to the suggestion that Ca^{2+}-dependent MLC phosphorylation may not be the only determinant of agonist-induced vascular tone and that the agonist may activate other mechanisms that increase the myofilament force sensitivity even in the absence of significant increases in $[Ca^{2+}]_i$ or MLC phosphorylation.

The mechanisms of the agonist-induced increase in the myofilament force sensitivity to Ca^{2+} and the second messengers involved have not been clearly identified. The interaction of an agonist with its receptor activates a GTP-binding protein, which activates the plasmalemmal enzyme phospholipase C, which in turn stimulates the hydrolysis of PIP_2 and increases the generation of the second messengers IP_3 and DAG [121] (see Figure 1.1). Another metabolic by-product of the agonist–receptor interaction is arachidonic acid, which can be produced from the hydrolysis of membrane phospholipids by phospholipase A_2 or from the transformation of DAG to arachidonic acid by DAG lipase. IP_3 stimulates Ca^{2+} release from intracellular stores and may explain the transient agonist-induced contraction in Ca^{2+}-free solution. Arachidonic acid at micromolar concentrations has been shown to inhibit MLC phosphatase suggesting its possible involvement in the agonist-induced increase in the myofilament force sensitivity to Ca^{2+}-dependent MLC phosphorylation [122]. On the other hand, DAG activates PKC. PKC is an ubiquitous enzyme that has been implicated in many cell functions including smooth muscle contraction.

·   ·   ·   ·   ·

CHAPTER 6

Protein Kinase C

Because of the small size and diffusible nature of Ca^{2+}, it has been feasible to envision its role in transducing the extracellular signal to the VSM contractile myofilaments. In contrast, the role of PKC in VSM contraction is not as widely perceived as Ca^{2+} partly because of its relatively large size, its numerous isoforms and substrates, and its differential subcellular distribution during VSM activation. Some important questions are how PKC is identified among other kinases in VSM and how the PKC signal is transferred from the receptors at the cell surface to the contractile myofilaments in the center of the cell. This section will discuss PKC structure, isoforms, protein substrates, subcellular distribution, and its potential role as a modulator of VSM function.

6.1   PKC STRUCTURE AND PKC ISOFORMS

PKC is an ubiquitous enzyme that was originally described as a Ca^{2+}-activated, phospholipid-dependent protein kinase [123]. Molecular cloning and biochemical analysis have revealed a family of PKC subspecies with closely related structures. The PKC isozymes α, β, and γ consist of four conserved (C1–C4) and five variable regions (V1–V5). The C1 region contains cysteine-rich zinc finger-like motifs that are immediately preceded by an autoinhibitory pseudosubstrate sequence and contains the recognition site for phosphatidylserine, DAG, and phorbol ester. The C2 region of some PKC isoforms is rich in acidic residues and contains the binding site for Ca^{2+}. The C3 and C4 regions constitute the ATP- and substrate-binding lobes of the PKC molecule [124–126] (Figure 6.1).

PKC isoforms are classified into three groups. The conventional PKCs α, βI, βII, and γ have the four conserved regions (C1–C4) and the five variable regions (V1–V5). The novel PKCs δ, ε, η(L), and θ lack the C2 region and therefore do not require Ca^{2+} for activation. The atypical PKCs ζ and λ/ι have only one cysteine-rich zinc finger-like motif and are dependent on phosphatidylserine, but not affected by DAG, phorbol esters, or Ca^{2+} (Figure 6.1).

6.2   PKC SUBSTRATES

When PKC is not catalytically active, the basic autoinhibitory pseudosubstrate is protected from proteolysis by an acidic patch in the substrate-binding site (Figure 6.2). When PKC is activated, it

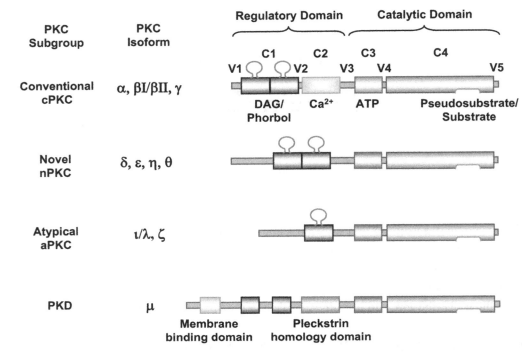

FIGURE 6.1: Structure of PKC isoforms. PKC is composed of four conserved (C1–C4) and five variable (V1–V5) regions. C1 region contains binding sites for DAG, phorbol ester, phosphatidylserine, and the PKC antagonist calphostin C. C2 region contains the binding site for Ca^{2+}. C3 and C4 regions contain binding sites for ATP, some PKC antagonists, and different PKC substrates. The PKC molecule folds to bring the ATP binding site into proximity with the substrate-binding site. Binding of an endogenous or exogenous pseudosubstrate peptide sequence to the catalytic domain prevents PKC from phosphorylating the true substrate.

phosphorylates arginine-rich protein substrates, which neutralize the acidic patch and displace the pseudosubstrate from its binding site in the kinase core [126,127]. The amino acid sequence near the substrate phosphorylation site may assist in PKC substrate recognition. PKC isotypes show specificity in substrate phosphorylation. While α-, β-, and γ-PKC are potent histone kinases, δ-, ε-, and η-PKC have a poor capacity to phosphorylate histone IIIS [125].

PKC causes phosphorylation of membrane-bound regulatory proteins in VSM. MARCKS (myristoylated, alanine-rich C kinase substrate), a major PKC substrate, is bound to F-actin and may function as a cross-bridge between cytoskeletal actin and the plasma membrane [128]. Also, PKC causes phosphorylation of the inhibitory GTP-binding protein G_i, facilitating the dissociation of the α_i subunit from adenylyl cyclase and thereby relieves it from inhibition [125].

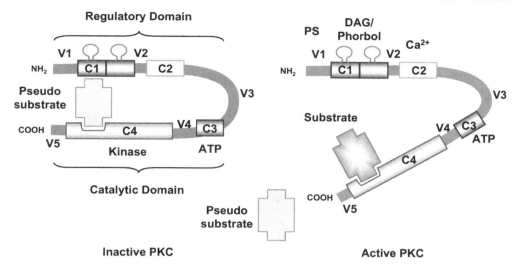

FIGURE 6.2: Mechanisms of PKC activation. The inactive PKC molecule is folded in such a way to have an endogenous pseudosubstare bind to the protein kinase region. PKC activation by phosphatidylserine (PS), DAG or phorbol ester, and Ca^{2+} allows the PKC molecule to unfold such that the true substrate can bind to the protein kinase region. In the presence of ATP, PKC causes phosphorylation of its true substrate.

PKC also affects plasma membrane channels and pumps. PKC inhibits BK_{Ca} channel activity in pulmonary VSM [129]. Also, thromboxane A_2-induced inhibition of voltage-gated K^+ channels and pulmonary vasoconstriction may involve ζ-PKC [130]. PKC may also phosphorylate and activate plasmalemmal or saroplasmic reticulum Ca^{2+}-ATPase, an action that promotes Ca^{2+} extrusion and may explain the transient nature of the agonist-induced increase in VSM $[Ca^{2+}]_i$. In addition, the $\alpha 1$ subunit of Na^+/K^+-ATPase may serve as a PKC substrate. Furthermore, activated PKC may phosphorylate and activate the Na^+/H^+ antiport exchanger and thereby increase the cytoplasmic pH [131].

PKC also phosphorylates regulatory proteins in VSM cytoskeleton and contractile myofilaments. PKC phosphorylates vinculin, a cytoskeletal protein localized at adhesion plaques, thus controlling cell shape and adhesion. PKC also phosphorylates CPI-17, which in turn inhibits MLC phosphatase, increases MLC phosphorylation, and thereby enhances VSM contraction [132]. The 20-kDa MLC and MLCK serve as substrates for PKC, and their phosphorylation could counteract the Ca^{2+}-induced actin–myosin interaction and force development [133]. On the other hand, activation of α-PKC could cause phosphorylation of calponin, an actin-associated regulatory protein, and thereby enhance VSM contraction [125]. A specific link likely exists between each PKC isoform and one or more specific substrates in VSM, and identification of these specific interactions needs to be further examined.

6.3 TISSUE DISTRIBUTION OF PKC

PKC isoforms are expressed in different proportions in VSM of various vascular beds (Table 6.1). α-PKC is a universal isoform that is expressed in almost all blood vessels tested. γ-PKC is mainly expressed in the neurons and vascular nerve endings. δ-PKC is mainly associated with the vascular cytoskeleton. ζ-PKC is a universal isoform that has been found in many tissues. η/L-PKC has been found in the lung, skin, heart, and brain. θ-PKC is mainly expressed in skeletal muscle, while ι/λ-PKC is expressed in the ovary and testis [125].

6.4 SUBCELLULAR DISTRIBUTION OF PKC

The PKC isoforms α, β, and γ are mainly localized in the cytosolic fraction of unstimulated cells and undergo translation to the cell membranes in activated cells (Table 6.1). δ-PKC is located almost exclusively in the particulate fraction of both resting and activated cells. While ζ-PKC is localized near the nucleus of resting and activated mature VSMCs [143], it could also play a role in pulmonary vasoconstriction in the perinatal period [144].

6.5 MECHANISMS OF PKC TRANSLOCATION

An important question is what causes PKC to translocate. Simple diffusion may provide the driving force, while targeting mechanisms could allow high-affinity binding when PKC is near its target [143]. Targeting mechanisms may involve one of the following:

6.5.1 Conformation-Induced Changes in Hydrophobicity

Binding of Ca^{2+} or DAG may cause conformational changes in the PKC molecule that could result in exposure of the pseudosubstrate region, increase the hydrophobicity of PKC, and facilitate its binding to membrane lipids [126].

6.5.2 Lipid Modification

Lipid modification of proteins changes their subcellular distribution. Myristoylation of MARCKS is required for its binding to actin at the plasma membrane. PKC-mediated phosphorylation of MARCKS causes its displacement from the membrane and interferes with its actin cross-linking. Dephosphorylation of MARCKS causes its reassociation with the membrane through its stably attached myristic acid membrane-targeting moiety [145].

TABLE 6.1: Subcellular Distribution of PKC

ENZYME	MOLECULAR WEIGHT (kDa)	CELL TYPE	RESTING STATE	ACTIVATED STATE	REFERENCE
PKC		Ferret portal vein	Cytosolic Perinuclear	Surface membrane Perinuclear	[134]
		Cultured rat aortic smooth muscle cells	Cytosolic fraction	Membrane fraction	[135]
α-PKC	74–82	Bovine aorta	Cytosolic fraction	Membrane fraction	[136]
		Ferret portal vein	Cytosolic fraction	Surface membrane	[137]
		Cultured rat aorta cells	Cytosolic fraction	Nuclear fraction	[138]
		Carotid artery	Cytosolic fraction	Particulate fraction	[139]
		Rat mesenteric artery	Cytosolic/ Membrane		[140]
β-PKC	80–82	Cultured rat aorta cells	Cytosolic fraction	Nuclear fraction	[138]
		Carotid artery	Cytosolic fraction	Particulate fraction	[139]
γ-PKC	70–82	Rat mesenteric artery	Cytosolic fraction	Cytosolic fraction	[140]
δ-PKC	76–82	Rat aorta	Cytoskeleton Organelles	Cytoskeleton Organelles	[141]

(continued on next page)

			TABLE 6.1: (continued)		
ENZYME	MOLECULAR WEIGHT (kDa)	CELL TYPE	RESTING STATE	ACTIVATED STATE	REFERENCE
		Rat mesenteric artery	Membrane fraction		[140]
ε-PKC	90–97	Ferret aorta	Cytosol	Surface membrane	[142]
		Rat mesenteric artery	Cytosolic/ Membrane		[140]
ζ-PKC	64–82	Ferret aorta and portal vein	Perinuclear	Intranuclear	[142]
		Rat aorta	Perinuclear	Intranuclear	[141]
		Rat mesenteric artery	Cytosolic fraction		[140]

The architecture of VSM plasma membrane appears to be regulated. VSM sarcolemma is divided into domains of focal adhesions alternating with caveolae-rich zones, both harboring a subset of membrane-associated proteins. Likewise, sarcolemmal lipids are segregated into domains of cholesterol-rich lipid rafts and glycerophospholipid-rich nonraft regions. The segregation of membrane lipids is critical for preservation of membrane protein architecture and for translocation of proteins to the sarcolemma. In smooth muscle, membrane lipid segregation is supported by annexins that target membrane sites of distinct lipid composition, and each annexin requires different $[Ca^{2+}]$ for its translocation to the sarcolemma, and thus allows a spatially confined, graded response to external stimuli and intracellular PKC [146].

6.5.3 Phosphorylation

The change in electric charge caused by phosphorylation of the protein may affect its affinity for lipid. For example, phosphorylation of MARCKS has an electrostatic effect of equal importance to myristoylation in determining the protein affinity to the membrane. Also, phosphorylation of PKC itself may be required for its activation and translocation. The PKC phosphorylation sites appear to be located in the catalytic domain of α-, β-, and δ-PKC [147].

6.5.4   Targeting Sequences

Binding sites for arginine-rich polypeptides have been identified in the PKC molecule distal to the catalytic site and may allow targeting of PKC to specific subcellular locations. Also, receptors for activated C-kinase (RACKs) may allow targeting of PKC to cytoskeletal elements, and a peptide inhibitor derived from the PKC-binding proteins annexin I and RACKI may interfere with translocation of p-PKC [148].

6.6   FUNCTIONS OF PKC IN VSM

PKC plays an important role in the cell adjustment to the environment by exerting both positive and negative effects on cellular events. PKC has been associated with numerous physiological functions, including secretion and exocytosis, modulation of ion conductance, gene expression, and cell proliferation [124,125]. PKC may also exert negative-feedback control over cell signaling via down-regulation of surface receptors and inhibition of agonist-mediated phosphoinositide hydrolysis [124]. Several studies suggest a role for PKC in VSM contraction [124,125,149–151]. PKC activation by phorbol esters has been shown to cause significant contraction in isolated vascular preparations [125,149]. Also, PKC inhibitors cause significant inhibition of agonist-induced vascular contraction [150,151]. However, some studies suggest that PKC-mediated phosphorylation of MLCK may cause vascular relaxation [133].

6.7   PKC ACTIVATORS

PKC isoforms respond differently to Ca^{2+}, phosphatidylserine, DAG, and other phospholipid degradation products. PKC binds Ca^{2+} in a phospholipid-dependent manner, and Ca^{2+} may form a "bridge" holding the protein and phospholipid complex together at the membrane [152]. Phosphatidylserine is indispensable for activation of PKC. Phosphatidylinositol and phosphatidic acid activate PKC at high Ca^{2+} concentrations. DAG activates PKC by reducing its Ca^{2+} requirement and enhancing its membrane association [124].

PKC activators also include lipids derived from sources other than glycerolipid hydrolysis such as cis-unsaturated free fatty acids and lysophosphatidylcholine, ceramide (a sphingomyelinase product), phosphatidylinositol 3,4,5-trisphosphate, and cholesterol sulfate [153]. Phorbol esters such as TPA, PMA, and PDBu can substitute for DAG in PKC activation. Phorbol esters stabilize PKC–membrane association by reducing its apparent K_m for Ca^{2+} [125].

Autophosphorylation of PKC may modify its activity or affinity for its substrates. α-, βI-, and βII-PKC are synthesized as inactive precursors that require phosphorylation by a putative "PKC kinase" for permissive activation. Also, multiple phosphorylation of α-PKC prevents its down-regulation by phorbol esters. Phosphorylation at the extreme C-terminus of βII-PKC allows the active site to bind ATP and substrate with higher affinity, while phosphorylation of structure determinants in the regulatory region enable higher affinity binding of Ca^{2+} [154].

6.8 PKC INHIBITORS

The role of PKC in VSM contraction has been verified by the use of PKC inhibitors. Several PKC inhibitors have been developed. PKC inhibitors acting in the catalytic domain compete with ATP and therefore may not be specific. PKC inhibitors acting in the regulatory domain compete at the DAG/phorbol ester or the phosphatidylserine binding site and may be more specific. Extended exposure to phorbol esters can specifically down-regulate α-, β-, and γ-PKC, but the tumor-promoting properties of phorbol esters limit their use.

The regulatory domain of PKC contains an amino acid sequence between residues 19 and 36 that resembles the substrate phosphorylation site. Synthetic oligopeptides based on pseudosubstrate sequence are specific PKC inhibitors because they exploit its substrate specificity and do not interfere with ATP binding. The synthetic peptide (19–36) inhibits both PKC autophosphorylation and protein substrate phosphorylation. Replacement of Arg-27 with alanine in the peptide [Ala-27]PKC (19–31) increases the IC_{50} for inhibition of substrate phosphorylation [127]. Also, a myristoylated peptide based on the substrate motif of α- and β-PKC, myr-ψPKC, inhibits TPA-Induced PKC activation and phosphorylation of MARCKS [155]. In smooth muscle, α-tocopherol inhibits the expression, activity, and phosphorylation of α-PKC. Interestingly, β-tocopherol protects PKC from the inhibitory effects of α-tocopherol [156].

siRNA for specific PKC isoforms is now available and should be useful for studying the role of PKC in various cell functions. Also, antisense techniques, transgenic animals, and knockout mice have been useful in studying the effects of PKC down-regulation in vivo.

6.9 PROTEIN KINASE CASCADES DURING VSM CONTRACTION

The interaction of a PKC isoform with its protein substrate may trigger a cascade of protein kinases that ultimately stimulate VSM contraction. PKC may phosphorylate CPI-17, which in turn inhibits MLC phosphatase, increases MLC phosphorylation, and enhances VSM contraction (see

Figure 1.1) [132]. PKC may also phosphorylate the actin-binding protein calponin, and thereby reverses its inhibition of actin-activated myosin ATPase, allows more actin to interact with myosin, and increases VSM contraction (Figure 1.1) [2].

PKC, MAPK, and c-Raf-1 have been implicated in VSM growth. MAPK is a Ser/Thr kinase that is activated by dual phosphorylation at Thr and Tyr residues. In quiescent undifferentiated cultured VSMCs, MAPK is mainly cytosolic but translocates to the nucleus during activation by mitogens. Tyrosine kinase and MAPK activities have also been identified in differentiated contractile VSM [143,157]. MAPK transiently translocates to the surface membrane during early activation of VSM but undergoes redistribution to the cytoskeleton during maintained VSM activation [157] (Figure 6.3). It has been suggested that during VSM activation, DAG promotes translocation of cytosolic ε-PKC to the surface membrane, where it is fully activated. Activated ε-PKC stimulates

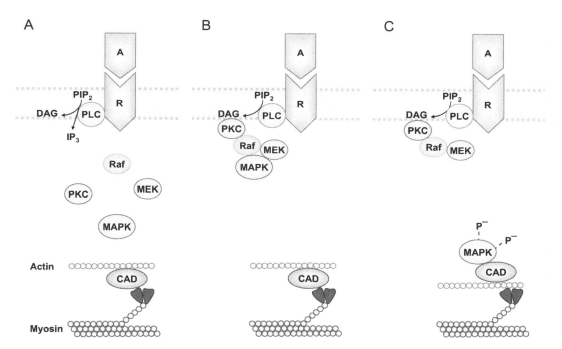

FIGURE 6.3: Protein kinase cascade leading to VSM contraction. Agonist (A)-induced activation of VSM receptor (R) leads to generation of DAG and translocation of PKC to the surface membrane (A). Other kinases such as Raf, MEK, and MAPK follow PKC and form a membrane complex (B). PKC via Raf and MEK leads to dual phosphorylation of MAPK. Phosphorylated MAPK undergoes redistribution to the core of the cell where it causes phosphorylation of the actin-binding protein caldesmon (CAD), allowing actin to interact with myosin and causing VSM contraction (C).

the translocation of cytosolic MEK and MAPK to the plasmalemma, where they form a surface membrane kinase complex. PKC causes phosphorylation and activation of MEK, which in turn phosphorylates MAPK at both Thr and Tyr residues. Tyrosine phosphorylation targets MAPK to the cytoskeleton, where it phosphorylates the actin-binding protein caldesmon and reverses its inhibition of MgATPase activity and thus increases actin–myosin interaction and VSM contraction (Figure 6.3) [2,157].

·   ·   ·   ·

CHAPTER 7

Rho Kinase in Vascular Smooth Muscle

Agonists of the G-protein-coupled receptors (GPCRs) such as phenylephrine, angiotensin II (AngII), and endothelin-1 (ET-1) stimulate phospholipase C and generate IP_3 and DAG. IP_3 activates receptors located on the sarcoplasmic reticulum, leading to Ca^{2+} release and a transient increase in $[Ca^{2+}]_i$. Agonists also stimulate Ca^{2+} entry through various types of Ca^{2+} channels leading to maintained increase in $[Ca^{2+}]_i$. Ca^{2+} then binds to CAM, and the resulting Ca^{2+}–CAM complex activates MLCK, which phosphorylates MLC, promoting the interaction of myosin with actin and subsequent VSM contraction. This mechanism of VSM contraction is entirely Ca^{2+}-dependent.

GPCR agonists, particularly those coupling to Ga12/13 proteins, can also activate the small G-protein RhoA. In its active GTP-bound form, RhoA activates Rho kinase (ROCK), which then phosphorylates and inactivates MLC phosphatase. This in turn increases the proportion of MLC in its phosphorylated form (MLC-P) and thereby promotes further VSM contraction. The ROCK-mediated enhancement of smooth muscle contraction occurs in the absence of significant changes in $[Ca^{2+}]_i$ and is therefore considered a Ca^{2+} sensitization mechanism [158–161].

7.1 ROCK STRUCTURE AND ISOFORMS

ROCKs are serine/threonine kinases with a molecular mass of ≈160 kDa. Two ROCK isoforms encoded by two different genes have been identified: ROCK-1 (ROCK I, or ROKβ) and ROCK-2 (ROCK II, or ROKα) [162–164]. Human ROCK-1 and ROCK-2 genes are located on chromosome 18 (18q11.1) and chromosome 2 (2p24), respectively. ROCK structure comprises a kinase domain located at the amino terminus of the protein, a coiled-coil region containing the Rho-binding domain, and a pleckstrin-homology domain with a cysteine-rich domain (Figure 7.1). ROCK-1 and ROCK-2 are highly homologous, with an overall amino acid sequence identity of 65%. The identity in the Rho-binding domain is 58% and approximately 92% in the kinase domain [165].

7.2 TISSUE EXPRESSION OF ROCK

Both ROCK-1 and ROCK-2 are ubiquitously expressed. ROCK-2 mRNA is highly expressed in the brain and skeletal muscle [165,166]. Both ROCK-1 and ROCK-2 are expressed in VSM and the heart [167].

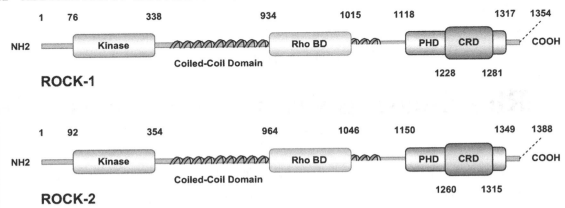

FIGURE 7.1: Molecular structure of ROCKs. ROCK amino acid sequence comprises a kinase domain located at the amino terminus, a coiled-coil region containing the Rho-binding domain (Rho BD), and a pleckstrin-homology domain (PHD) with a cysteine-rich domain (CRD). ROCK-1 and ROCK-2 are highly homologous with an overall amino acid sequence identity of 65%.

Some studies suggest that the expression of ROCK is regulated. Both ROCK-1 and ROCK-2 mRNAs and proteins are up-regulated by AngII via angiotensin type 1 receptor stimulation and by interleukin-1β [168]. The up-regulation of ROCK may occur through PKC- and nuclear factor κB-dependent pathways. Also, chronic administration of AngII in mice is associated with up-regulation of ROCK in coronary artery [168].

7.3 SUBCELLULAR DISTRIBUTION OF ROCK

Similar to other GTPases, Rho cycles between an inactive guanosine diphosphate (GDP)-bound form and an active GTP-bound form. When bound to GTP, Rho recognizes and interacts with its downstream targets and initiates a cellular response. The subcellular localization of Rho also determines its activation state. In unstimulated cells, RhoA resides predominantly in the cytosol, bound to GDP. During receptor stimulation, RhoA undergoes translocation to the plasma membrane where GDP–GTP exchange takes place [161]. The translocation of RhoA to the plasma membrane is facilitated by the hydrophobic geranylgeranyl tail that is attached to the C-terminal of RhoA during posttranslational modification of the protein.

ROCKs are also essentially distributed in the cytoplasm but are partially translocated to peripheral membrane during RhoA activation [163,164]. The mechanisms responsible for the subcellular localization of ROCKs are unclear but could involve mechanisms involved in the translocation of other protein kinases such as PKC.

7.4   REGULATION OF ROCK ACTIVITY

The C-terminal of ROCK contains an autoinhibitory region [169], including the pleckstrin-homology and Rho-binding domains (Figure 7.2). Each of these domains binds independently to the N-terminal kinase domain and, in turn, inhibits the enzyme activity [170]. During ROCK activation, the interaction between the C-terminal autoinhibitory region and kinase domain is disrupted. This disruption could occur as a result of binding of RhoA or complete cleavage of the C-terminal, which yields a constitutively active kinase.

The kinase domain of ROCKs is localized in the N-terminal region of the protein sequence. Truncated forms of ROCKs lacking the C-terminal portion of the protein, which contains the Rho-binding domain and the pleckstrin-homology domain, are constitutively active, whereas C-terminal portions of ROCKs expressed in cells act as dominant negatives [171]. This led to the suggestion that the C-terminal region of ROCKs is a negative regulatory region, responsible for autoinhibition of the kinase activity in resting cells, probably through interaction with the catalytic domain of ROCKs [172]. Oligomerization (dimerization) also influences the kinase activity of ROCKs and its affinity for ATP [173]. Binding of active GTP-bound form of RhoA to Rho-binding domain stimulates the phosphotransferase activity of ROCK by disrupting the interaction between the catalytic and the inhibitory C-terminal region of the enzyme. However, the stimulatory effect of GTP-RhoA on the enzyme activity of ROCKs is limited to a 1.5- to 2-fold increase [174]. Lipids such as arachidonic acid or sphingosine phosphorylcholine efficiently increase ROCK activity 5- to 6-fold independently of RhoA [174,175]. Arachidonic acid and sphingosine phosphorylcholine

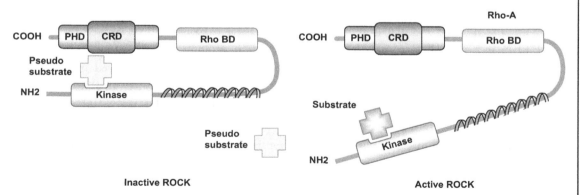

FIGURE 7.2: Mechanisms of ROCK activation. In the inactive form, the C terminus of ROCK is folded over the N-terminal region of the enzyme, forming an autoinhibitory loop. Binding of active GTP-bound RhoA causes unfolding and activation of ROCKs, and thereby exposes the kinase domain and allows phosphorylation of the true substrate.

may interact with the regulatory region of ROCK, possibly the pleckstrin-homology domain, thus disrupting its inhibitory action on the catalytic activity of ROCK [172]. ROCKs are also activated by cleavage of the inhibitory C-terminal region, which results in the release of a truncated active form of the kinase.

Negative control of the kinase activity of ROCKs has also been described. The small G-protein RhoE binds to the N-terminal region of ROCK-1 (amino acids 1–420) containing the kinase domain [176]. RhoE binding to ROCK-1 inhibits its activity and prevents RhoA binding to Rho-binding domain [176]. Two other small G proteins, Gem and Rad, have been shown to bind and inhibit ROCK function, but their mechanism of action is not clear [177].

7.5   ROCK SUBSTRATES

The consensus sequence of ROCK phosphorylation site is RXXS/T or RXS/T [178–181]. ROCKs seem to require basic amino acids such as Arg (R) close to its phosphorylation site. More than 15 ROCK substrates have been identified. For many ROCK substrates, the functional consequence of ROCK-mediated phosphorylation is related to actin filament formation and organization and cytoskeleton rearrangements [182,183].

A major group of ROCK targets includes the myosin phosphatase target subunit (MYPT-1) [184], CPI-17 [185], the 20-kDa MLC [178], and calponin [186], which are known to modulate smooth muscle cell contraction. MYPT-1 is the major effector of ROCK-mediated Ca^{2+} sensitization pathway of smooth muscle contraction. Cardiac troponin is another ROCK substrate. Phosphorylation of troponin by ROCK causes reduction in tension generation in cardiac myocytes [187].

Phosphatase and tensin homologue (PTEN) is a newly identified ROCK substrate [188]. PTEN is a phosphatase that dephosphorylates both proteins and phosphoinositide substrates such as the phosphatidylinositol 3-kinase (PI_3-kinase)/Akt pathway involved in the regulation of cell growth, protein synthesis, transcriptional regulation, and cell survival. Phosphorylation of PTEN by ROCK stimulates its phosphatase activity, and ROCK inhibitors could reduce ROCK-mediated PTEN phosphorylation and thereby enhances Akt signaling in endothelial cells [189]. Active ROCK also interacts with and phosphorylates the insulin receptor substrate-1 (IRS-1) in VSMCs, leading to inhibition of both insulin-induced IRS-1 tyrosine phosphorylation and PI_3-kinase activation [190]. In VSMCs from hypertensive rats, the ROCK/IRS-1 association is increased, and insulin signaling is markedly reduced [190].

Most of ROCK substrates have been identified from in vitro experiments performed after either activation of endogenous ROCK or transfection of one of the two ROCK isoforms. Because the kinase domains of both isoforms are nearly identical, it has been thought that ROCK-1 and ROCK-2 share the same substrates. However, ROCK-1 but not ROCK-2 binds to and phosphorylates RhoE, providing evidence that ROCK-1 and ROCK-2 have different targets [191]. The N-terminal regions, upstream of the kinase domains of ROCKs, are involved in the interaction with the substrates [176] and could play a role in determining substrate specificity of the ROCK isoforms.

7.6   ROCK AND VSM FUNCTION

A large body of evidence suggests important functions of ROCK in VSMCs. The phosphorylation/dephosphorylation of MLC is a major regulatory mechanism of smooth muscle contraction. A rise in $[Ca^{2+}]_i$ causes activation of MLCK and consequent phosphorylation of MLC and smooth muscle contraction. However, MLC phosphorylation and VSM contraction can be induced in the absence of significant increases in $[Ca^{2+}]_i$. RhoA-mediated ROCK activation phosphorylates MYPT-1, the regulatory subunit of MLC phosphatase, and inhibits its activity and thereby causes Ca^{2+} sensitization of the contractile proteins and enhances VSM contraction.

ROCK is not only a major regulator of VSM cell contraction but is also important in controlling cell migration, proliferation, apoptosis/survival, gene transcription, and differentiation.

To investigate the role of ROCK isoforms in vivo, ROCK-1 and ROCK-2 knockout mice have been generated. ROCK-1-deficient mice have open eyelids at birth [192]. ROCK-2-deficient mice develop placental dysfunction leading to intrauterine growth retardation and fetal death [193]. The cardiovascular phenotype of ROCK-1 and ROCK-2 knockout mice has not been clearly analyzed.

7.7   RHO KINASE INHIBITORS

ROCK activation involves RhoA translocation to the plasma membrane, RhoA binding to ROCK, and ATP-dependent phosphorylation of various substrates. Interference with any of these processes could inhibit ROCK activity, phosphorylation of the specific substrate, and inhibition of ROCK-stimulated cellular response. For example, disruption of the prenylation process, by agents such as 3-hydroxy-3-methylglutaryl-coenzyme A reductase inhibitors (statins) or protein prenyltransferase inhibitors, can prevent the membrane translocation and activation of Rho and thereby impair the ability of Rho to activate its downstream target ROCK. Some pharmacological ROCK inhibitors exert their effect by competing with ATP for binding at the kinase domain, or "active site" of the enzyme. Some of the commonly known ROCK inhibitors include Y-27632 and fasudil.

Y-27632 is a synthetic pyridine derivative that inhibits ROCK by competing with ATP for the kinase active site. Y-27632 has an affinity for ROCK that is ~200- and ~2000-fold higher than for the structurally similar kinases PKC and MLCK, respectively. Y-27632 selectively lower elevated blood pressure in animal models of experimental hypertension, supporting a link between

VSM ROCK and the development of hypertension [194]. Experiments with Y-27632 have also revealed that ROCK activity might be enhanced in the cerebral circulation under conditions of chronic hypertension [195–198]. These experimental findings made Y-27632 a promising candidate as a potential therapeutic antihypertensive agent. However, despite its utility in numerous experimental studies in vivo [194,199,200], the safety profile of Y-27632 has not yet been verified and its future use as a therapeutic agent is uncertain.

In addition to its ability to potently inhibit ROCKI and ROCKII, Y-27632 could inhibit PKC-related kinase (PRK2) with a similar potency to that of ROCKII [201], although the role of PRK2 in the vasculature is unknown. Also, at a high 10-μM concentration, Y-27632 inhibits PKC-dependent vasoconstriction [202]. Although these observations suggest that ROCK activation may occur downstream of PKC-mediated vasoconstriction as have been described in the coronary circulation [203], the possibility that Y-27632 causes nonselective inhibition of PKC cannot be ruled out.

Fasudil is an isoquinoline derivative that also inhibits ROCK by competing with ATP for the kinase active site. Fasudil has been used to characterize the role of ROCK in vascular function in small-scale clinical studies [204–206]. The good safety profile of fasudil has facilitated its approval for use in Japan for the treatment of cerebral vasospasm following subarachnoid hemorrhage. After oral administration, fasudil is metabolized to the more selective ROCK inhibitor hydroxyfasudil. Hence, fasudil is thought of as a prodrug whose therapeutic effects stem from the relatively potent and selective ROCK inhibitor activity of its metabolite.

It is important to note that the active site of ROCK is similar to that of protein kinase A (PKA), the target of cyclic adenosine monophosphate that mediates vasodilation and inhibits platelet aggregation. This structural similarity may account for the ability of fasudil to inhibit ROCK and PKA with equal potency [207] and raise the possibility of unwanted effects in the clinical use of fasudil as a result of PKA inhibition. Although the metabolite hydroxyfasudil is 15-fold more selective for ROCK than for PKA [207], the possibility that fasudil may exert unwanted vascular effects if its metabolism was compromised should be taken into account. Studies have revealed important sequence differences between ROCK and PKA, which could be used to further improve the selectivity of future ROCK inhibitors [207].

C H A P T E R   8

Vascular Smooth Muscle Dysfunction and Vascular Disease

The signaling mechanisms of VSM contraction are altered in pathological vascular conditions. Systemic hypertension is characterized by high arterial pressure partly due to increased vascular resistance as a result of enhanced VSM contractility and arterial wall remodeling. An increase in plasma membrane permeability to Ca^{2+} and increased $[Ca^{2+}]_i$ have been demonstrated in VSMCs isolated from animal models of hypertension and coronary vasospasm [208–210]. These observations have suggested the use of Ca^{2+} channel blockers for treatment of these cardiovascular disorders. However, Ca^{2+} antagonist-insensitive forms of hypertension and coronary vasospasm have been demonstrated, and a role for other factors in addition to the elevation of $[Ca^{2+}]_i$ in these vascular diseases has been suggested.

PKC has been suggested to play a role in the pathogenesis of coronary and cerebral vasospasm, hypertension, hypertensive medial hypertrophy, atherogenesis, and microvascular and macrovascular complications of diabetes [3,211,212]. These vascular disorders are characterized by increased contractile or hypertrophic response of VSMCs due to increased production of or sensitivity to vasoconstrictive stimuli and vascular growth factors. Many of these stimuli, including AngII, vasopressin, norepinephrine, and platelet-derived growth factor, bind to receptors that trigger a G-protein-mediated activation of phospholipase C [18,213] causing the generation of DAG, a physiological activator of PKC.

High-fat diets in general appear to increase PKC activity and cause adverse cardiovascular consequences. However, long-chain omega-3 polyunsaturates from fish oil may limit PKC activation under certain conditions. Fish oil-rich diets tend to reduce elevated blood pressure [214] and the vasoconstrictive response to AngII and norepinephrine in humans [215]. These effects are likely due to decreased DAG production and PKC activity because preincubation of rat VSMCs with eicosapentaenoic acid prevents vasopressin-mediated increase in membrane content of DAG [216].

Each PKC isoform appears to have a peculiar tissue or cellular distribution, a specific substrate, and thereby a specific cellular function. For instance, α-PKC may play a role in Ca^{2+}-dependent contraction of VSM [137] and overexpression of α-PKC has been implicated in the pathogenesis of hypertension [141]. The subcellular distribution of each PKC isoform may also be critical for normal cell function. In normotensive rats, α-PKC is localized mainly in the cytosol of VSMCs. α-PKC appears to be hyperactivated and concentrated at the cell membrane of VSMCs in hypertensive animals [141].

Treatment of a PKC-mediated pathological condition would require selective inhibition of the expression or activity of a specific PKC isoform. Knockout animal models that lack a specific PKC isoform have been developed. Also, potent pharmacological tools that specifically inhibit one PKC subspecies have been designed. The first generation of PKC antagonists has not been very selective. While some of the new PKC antagonists appear to be more selective, rigorous laboratory experiments are needed before they can be safely used in humans.

The ROCK inhibitors Y-27632 and fasudil normalize arterial pressure in animal models of hypertension indicating the importance of the ROCK signaling pathway in the vascular hyper-reactivity associated with hypertension [194]. Measurements of the amount of active GTP-bound RhoA in arteries from animal models of hypertension have shown an increased RhoA activity and enhanced ROCK activation [217]. Also, chronic inhibition of ROCK suppresses vascular medial hypertrophy and perivascular fibrosis in coronary arteries of spontaneously hypertensive rats [218] and in a rat model of hypertension induced by chronic inhibition of nitric oxide synthesis [219]. In both models, the activity of RhoA/ROCK pathway is increased. Also, inhibition of angiotensin type 1 receptor decreases RhoA/ROCK activity, suggesting that the activation of ROCK in hypertensive rats is likely due to an increase in AngII activity [219]. This is supported by report that long-term infusion of AngII increases the activity of RhoA and ROCK and increases medial thickness and perivascular fibrosis in coronary arteries, and AngII-induced coronary hypertrophy and fibrosis are inhibited by ROCK inhibitors [220]. ROCK inhibition is also associated with reduction of AngII-induced production of superoxide anion [220], monocyte chemoattractant protein-1, and PAI-1 [221,222]. Also, in hypertension, mechanical strain on the vessel wall is increased and mechanical stress stimulates VSMC proliferation [223]. In effect, stretch-induced activation of MAPK and VSMC growth are inhibited by ROCK inhibition [224,225]. Excessive RhoA/ROCK activity could also participate in the endothelial dysfunction and the decreased nitric oxide production associated with arterial diseases. Together, these findings point to a prominent role of ROCKs in hypertension.

Pulmonary hypertension is a multifactorial disorder that involves sustained vasoconstriction and structural remodeling of pulmonary arteries leading to reduction of the lumen area of the pulmonary microvasculature and elevation of pulmonary vascular resistance. Reduced endothelium-derived nitric oxide production in pulmonary arteries has been implicated in the pathophysiology of pulmonary hypertension [226]. Studies on human pulmonary endothelial cells demonstrated that hypoxia-induced decrease in eNOS expression is mediated by ROCK [227]. Studies have also shown that activation of the RhoA/ROCK pathway contributes to both vasoconstriction and vascular remodeling associated with pulmonary hypertension [228,229]. The ROCK inhibitor

Y-27632 attenuates acute hypoxia-induced vasoconstriction and reduces the development of chronic hypoxia-induced pulmonary hypertension and vascular remodeling [230]. Also, chronic hypoxia in rats is associated with 2-fold increase in ROCK expression and enhanced ROCK-dependent Ca^{2+} sensitization in small pulmonary arteries [231]. The ROCK pathway is also involved in monocrotaline-induced pulmonary hypertension in rats, and long-term inhibition of ROCK by oral or inhaled fasudil improves monocrotaline-induced pulmonary hypertension as a result of inhibition of VSMC proliferation and increased apoptosis, reduced macrophage infiltration, and improved endothelium-dependent pulmonary artery relaxation [229,232,233]. These findings indicate that activation of the RhoA/ROCK pathway is involved in the pathogenesis of pulmonary hypertension, although the mechanisms leading to the increased RhoA/ROCK activity are unclear.

. . . .

CHAPTER 9

Summary

Ca^{2+} is a major determinant of VSM functions. $[Ca^{2+}]_i$ is controlled by two opposing Ca^{2+} handling mechanisms composed of Ca^{2+} channels and Ca^{2+} pumps in the plasma membrane and intracellular organelles. Ca^{2+} mobilizing mechanisms tend to increase $[Ca^{2+}]_i$ while the Ca^{2+} homeostatic mechanisms have the opposite effect. The balance between the Ca^{2+} mobilizing and the Ca^{2+} homeostatic mechanisms maintains resting $[Ca^{2+}]_i$ constant. In the presence of a physiological agonist or in pathological states such as hypertension, the balance between the Ca^{2+} mobilizing and the Ca^{2+} homeostatic mechanisms is compromised leading to an increase in $[Ca^{2+}]_i$ and VSM contraction.

Interaction of an agonist with its plasma membrane receptor elevates the cellular level of two second messengers. The first is $[Ca^{2+}]_i$ by stimulating Ca^{2+} release from intracellular stores and Ca^{2+} influx from extracellular space. The second is DAG by stimulating the hydrolysis of PIP_2 and phosphatidylcholine. The increase in $[Ca^{2+}]_i$ activates the Ca^{2+}-dependent MLC phosphorylation pathway and initiates the development of force. The maintained increase in DAG activates PKC, and activated PKC may translocate to cellular membranes. The PKC catalytic domain may relocate to the cell interior to phosphorylate cytoplasmic substrates, a process that increases the myofilament force sensitivity to Ca^{2+} and enhances VSM contraction. PKC isoforms exhibit different tissue- and cell type-specific expression patterns, suggesting a specific subcellular location, substrate, and function for each PKC isoform. Agonists could also increase the activity of ROCK leading to inhibition of MLC phosphatase and further enhancement of the myofilament force sensitivity to Ca^{2+}. Concomitant increases in $[Ca^{2+}]_i$, PKC and ROCK activity may promote vasoconstriction, VSM hypertrophy and hyperplasia, and the vascular remodeling associated with vascular disease.

· · · · ·

References

[1]   Khalil RA, van Breemen C. Mechanisms of calcium mobilization and homeostasis in vascular smooth muscle and their relevance to hypertension. In: Laragh JH, Brenner BM, eds. *Hypertension: Pathophysiology, Diagnosis and Management*, 2nd ed. New York, NY: Raven Press Publishers; 1995, pp. 523–40.

[2]   Kim HR, Appel S, Vetterkind S, Gangopadhyay SS, Morgan KG. Smooth muscle signalling pathways in health and disease, *J Cell Mol Med*, 2008;12(6A):2165–80.

[3]   Salamanca DA, Khalil RA. Protein kinase C isoforms as specific targets for modulation of vascular smooth muscle function in hypertension, *Biochem Pharmacol*, 2005;70(11): pp. 1537–47.

[4]   Somlyo AP, Somlyo AV. Signal transduction by G-proteins, rho-kinase and protein phosphatase to smooth muscle and non-muscle myosin II, *J Physiol*, 2000;522(Pt 2): pp. 177–85.

[5]   Khalil RA, van Breemen C. Sustained contraction of vascular smooth muscle: calcium influx or C-kinase activation? *J Pharmacol Exp Ther*, 1988;244(2): pp. 537–42.

[6]   Cauvin C, Loutzenhiser R, Van Breemen C. Mechanisms of calcium antagonist-induced vasodilation, *Annu Rev Pharmacol Toxicol*, 1983;23: pp. 373–96.

[7]   Deth R, van Breemen C. Agonist induced release of intracellular Ca^{2+} in the rabbit aorta, *J Membr Biol*, 1977;30(4): pp. 363–80.

[8]   Somlyo AP, Somlyo AV. Smooth muscle structure and function. In: Fozzard HA, Haber E, Jennings RB, Katz AM, Morgan HE, eds. *The Heart and Cardiovascular System*, 2nd ed, New York, NY: Raven Press Publishers; 1992, pp. 1295–1324.

[9]   Endo M. Calcium release from the sarcoplasmic reticulum, *Physiol Rev*, 1977;57(1): pp. 71–108.

[10] Devine CE, Somlyo AV, Somlyo AP. Sarcoplasmic reticulum and mitochondria as cation accumulation sites in smooth muscle, *Philos Trans R Soc Lond B Biol Sci*, 1973;265: pp. 17–23.

[11] Bond M, Kitazawa T, Somlyo AP, Somlyo AV. Release and recycling of calcium by the sarcoplasmic reticulum in guinea-pig portal vein smooth muscle, *J Physiol*, 1984;355: pp. 677–95.

[12] Ehrlich BE, Watras J. Inositol 1,4,5-trisphosphate activates a channel from smooth muscle sarcoplasmic reticulum, *Nature*, 1988;336(6199): pp. 583–86.

[13] Saida K, Van Breemen C. Cyclic AMP modulation of adrenoreceptor-mediated arterial smooth muscle contraction, *J Gen Physiol*, 1984;84(2): pp. 307–18.

[14] Cassidy P, Hoar PE, Kerrick WG. Irreversible thiophosphorylation and activation of tension in functionally skinned rabbit ileum strips by [35S]ATP gamma S, *J Biol Chem*, 1979; 254(21): pp. 11148–53.

[15] Nishimura J, Kolber M, van Breemen C. Norepinephrine and GTP-gamma-S increase myofilament Ca^{2+} sensitivity in alpha-toxin permeabilized arterial smooth muscle, *Biochem Biophys Res Commun*, 1988;157(2): pp. 677–83.

[16] Kitazawa T, Kobayashi S, Horiuti K, Somlyo AV, Somlyo AP. Receptor-coupled, permeabilized smooth muscle. Role of the phosphatidylinositol cascade, G-proteins, and modulation of the contractile response to Ca^{2+}, *J Biol Chem*, 1989;264(10): pp. 5339–42.

[17] Berridge MJ, Irvine RF. Inositol trisphosphate, a novel second messenger in cellular signal transduction, *Nature*, 1984;312(5992): pp. 315–21.

[18] Griendling KK, Rittenhouse SE, Brock TA, Ekstein LS, Gimbrone MA Jr, Alexander RW. Sustained diacylglycerol formation from inositol phospholipids in angiotensin II-stimulated vascular smooth muscle cells, *J Biol Chem*, 1986;261(13): pp. 5901–06.

[19] Suematsu E, Hirata M, Hashimoto T, Kuriyama H. Inositol 1,4,5-trisphosphate releases Ca^{2+} from intracellular store sites in skinned single cells of porcine coronary artery, *Biochem Biophys Res Commun*, 1984;120(2): pp. 481–85.

[20] Somlyo AV, Bond M, Somlyo AP, Scarpa A. Inositol trisphosphate-induced calcium release and contraction in vascular smooth muscle, *Proc Natl Acad Sci* USA, 1985;82(15): pp. 5231–35.

[21] Yamamoto H, van Breemen C. Inositol-1,4,5-trisphosphate releases calcium from skinned cultured smooth muscle cells, *Biochem Biophys Res Commun*, 1985;130(1): pp. 270–74.

[22] Saida K, van Breemen C. GTP requirement for inositol-1,4,5-trisphosphate-induced Ca^{2+} release from sarcoplasmic reticulum in smooth muscle, *Biochem Biophys Res Commun*, 1987;144(3): pp. 1313–16.

[23] Iino M. Calcium dependent inositol trisphosphate-induced calcium release in the guinea-pig taenia caeci, *Biochem Biophys Res Commun*, 1987;142(1): pp. 47–52.

[24] Walker JW, Somlyo AV, Goldman YE, Somlyo AP, Trentham DR. Kinetics of smooth and skeletal muscle activation by laser pulse photolysis of caged inositol 1,4,5-trisphosphate, *Nature*, 1987;327(6119): pp. 249–52.

[25] Kobayashi S, Somlyo AV, Somlyo AP. Heparin inhibits the inositol 1,4,5-trisphosphate-dependent, but not the independent, calcium release induced by guanine nucleotide in vascular smooth muscle, *Biochem Biophys Res Commun*, 1988;153(2): pp. 625–31.

[26] Ford LE, Podolsky RJ. Regenerative calcium release within muscle cells, *Science*, 1970; 167(914): pp. 58–59.

[27] Fabiato A, Fabiato F. Excitation–contraction coupling of isolated cardiac fibers with disrupted or closed sarcolemmas. Calcium-dependent cyclic and tonic contractions, *Circ Res*, 1972;31(3): pp. 293–307.

[28] van Breemen C, Saida K. Cellular mechanisms regulating $[Ca^{2+}]_i$ smooth muscle, *Annu Rev Physiol*, 1989;51: pp. 315–29.

[29] Benham CD, Tsien RW. A novel receptor-operated Ca^{2+}-permeable channel activated by ATP in smooth muscle, *Nature*, 1987;328(6127): pp. 275–78.

[30] Van Breemen C. Calcium requirement for activation of intact aortic smooth muscle, *J Physiol*, 1977;272(2): pp. 317–29.

[31] Bean BP, Sturek M, Puga A, Hermsmeyer K. Calcium channels in muscle cells isolated from rat mesenteric arteries: modulation by dihydropyridine drugs, *Circ Res*, 1986;59(2): pp. 229–35.

[32] Loirand G, Pacaud P, Mironneau C, Mironneau J. Evidence for two distinct calcium channels in rat vascular smooth muscle cells in short-term primary culture, *Pflügers Arch*, 1986;407(5): pp. 566–68.

[33] Benham CD, Hess P, Tsien RW. Two types of calcium channels in single smooth muscle cells from rabbit ear artery studied with whole-cell and single-channel recordings, *Circ Res*, 1987;61(4 Pt 2): pp. 110–16.

[34] Yatani A, Seidel CL, Allen J, Brown AM. Whole-cell and single-channel calcium currents of isolated smooth muscle cells from saphenous vein, *Circ Res*, 1987;60(4): pp. 523–33.

[35] Bolton TB. Mechanisms of action of transmitters and other substances on smooth muscle, *Physiol Rev*, 1979;59(3): pp. 606–718.

[36] Van Breemen C, Aaronson P, Loutzenhiser R. Sodium–calcium interactions in mammalian smooth muscle, *Pharmacol Rev*, 1978;30(2): pp. 167–208.

[37] Nelson MT, Standen NB, Brayden JE, Worley JF 3rd. Noradrenaline contracts arteries by activating voltage-dependent calcium channels, *Nature*, 1988;336(6197): pp. 382–85.

[38] Sturek M, Hermsmeyer K. Calcium and sodium channels in spontaneously contracting vascular muscle cells, *Science*, 1986;233(4762): pp. 475–78.

[39] Benham CD, Tsien RW. Noradrenaline modulation of calcium channels in single smooth muscle cells from rabbit ear artery, *J Physiol*, 1988;404: pp. 767–84.

[40] Meisheri KD, Hwang O, van Breemen C. Evidence for two separated Ca^{2+} pathways in smooth muscle plasmalemma, *J Membr Biol*, 1981;59(1): pp. 19–25.

[41] Reuter H. Modulation of ion channels by phosphorylation and second messengers, *News Physiol Sci*, 1987;2: pp. 168–71.

[42] Putney JW Jr. TRP, inositol 1,4,5-trisphosphate receptors, and capacitative calcium entry, *Proc Natl Acad Sci* USA, 1999;96(26): pp. 14669–71.

[43] Putney JW Jr. Pharmacology of capacitative calcium entry, *Mol Interv*, 2001;1(2): pp. 84–94.

[44] Leung FP, Yung LM, Yao X, Laher I, Huang Y. Store-operated calcium entry in vascular smooth muscle, *Br J Pharmacol*, 2008;153(5): pp. 846–57.

[45] Parekh AB, Putney JW Jr. Store-operated calcium channels, *Physiol Rev*, 2005;85(2): pp. 757–810.

[46] Hoth M, Penner R. Depletion of intracellular calcium stores activates a calcium current in mast cells, *Nature*, 1992;355(6358): pp. 353–56.

[47] Parekh AB. Functional consequences of activating store-operated CRAC channels, *Cell Calcium*, 2007;42(2): pp. 111–21.

[48] Xuan YT, Wang OL, Whorton AR. Thapsigargin stimulates Ca^{2+} entry in vascular smooth muscle cells: nicardipine-sensitive and -insensitive pathways, *Am J Physiol*, 1992;262(5 Pt 1): pp. C1258–65.

[49] Xuan YT, Glass PS. Propofol regulation of calcium entry pathways in cultured A10 and rat aortic smooth muscle cells, *Br J Pharmacol*, 1996;117(1): pp. 5–12.

[50] Tosun M, Paul RJ, Rapoport RM. Coupling of store-operated Ca^{++} entry to contraction in rat aorta, *J Pharmacol Exp Ther*, 1998;285(2): pp. 759–66.

[51] Smani T, Zakharov SI, Csutora P, Leno E, Trepakova ES, Bolotina VM. A novel mechanism for the store-operated calcium influx pathway, *Nat Cell Biol*, 2004;6(2): pp. 113–20.

[52] Trepakova ES, Gericke M, Hirakawa Y, Weisbrod RM, Cohen RA, Bolotina VM. Properties of a native cation channel activated by Ca^{2+} store depletion in vascular smooth muscle cells, *J Biol Chem*, 2001;276(11): pp. 7782–90.

[53] Kim HY, Thomas D, Hanley MR. Chromatographic resolution of an intracellular calcium influx factor from thapsigargin-activated Jurkat cells. Evidence for multiple activities influencing calcium elevation in *Xenopus* oocytes, *J Biol Chem*, 1995;270(17): pp. 9706–08.

[54] Golovina VA, Platoshyn O, Bailey CL, Wang J, Limsuwan A, Sweeney M, Rubin LJ, Yuan JX. Upregulated TRP and enhanced capacitative Ca^{2+} entry in human pulmonary artery myocytes during proliferation, *Am J Physiol Heart Circ Physiol*, 2001;280(2): pp. H746–55.

[55] Xu SZ, Beech DJ. TrpC1 is a membrane-spanning subunit of store-operated Ca^{2+} channels in native vascular smooth muscle cells, *Circ Res*, 2001;88(1): pp. 84–87.

[56] Bergdahl A, Gomez MF, Wihlborg AK, Erlinge D, Eyjolfson A, Xu SZ, Beech DJ, Dreja K, Hellstrand P. Plasticity of TRPC expression in arterial smooth muscle: correlation with store-operated Ca^{2+} entry, *Am J Physiol Cell Physiol*, 2005;288(4): pp. C872–80.

[57] Giamarchi A, Padilla F, Coste B, Raoux M, Crest M, Honoré E, Delmas P. The versatile nature of the calcium-permeable cation channel TRPP2, *EMBO Rep*, 2006;7(8): pp. 787–93.

[58]   Xu SZ, Boulay G, Flemming R, Beech DJ. E3-targeted anti-TRPC5 antibody inhibits store-operated calcium entry in freshly isolated pial arterioles, *Am J Physiol Heart Circ Physiol*, 2006;291(6): pp. H2653–59.

[59]   Strübing C, Krapivinsky G, Krapivinsky L, Clapham DE. Formation of novel TRPC channels by complex subunit interactions in embryonic brain, *J Biol Chem*, 2003;278(40): pp. 39014–19.

[60]   Zagranichnaya TK, Wu X, Villereal ML. Endogenous TRPC1, TRPC3, and TRPC7 proteins combine to form native store-operated channels in HEK-293 cells, *J Biol Chem*, 2005;280(33): pp. 29559–69.

[61]   Roos J, DiGregorio PJ, Yeromin AV, Ohlsen K, Lioudyno M, Zhang S, Safrina O, Kozak JA, Wagner SL, Cahalan MD, Veliçelebi G, Stauderman KA. STIM1, an essential and conserved component of store-operated Ca^{2+} channel function, *J Cell Biol*, 2005;169(3): pp. 435–45.

[62]   López JJ, Salido GM, Pariente JA, Rosado JA. Interaction of STIM1 with endogenously expressed human canonical TRP1 upon depletion of intracellular Ca^{2+} stores, *J Biol Chem*, 2006;281(38): pp. 28254–64.

[63]   Prakriya M, Feske S, Gwack Y, Srikanth S, Rao A, Hogan PG. Orai1 is an essential pore subunit of the CRAC channel, *Nature*, 2006;443(7108): pp. 230–33.

[64]   Navarro-Borelly L, Somasundaram A, Yamashita M, Ren D, Miller RJ, Prakriya M. STIM1-Orai1 interactions and Orai1 conformational changes revealed by live-cell FRET microscopy, *J Physiol*, 2008;586(Pt 22): pp. 5383–401.

[65]   Soboloff J, Spassova MA, Tang XD, Hewavitharana T, Xu W, Gill DL. Orai1 and STIM reconstitute store-operated calcium channel function, *J Biol Chem*, 2006;281(30): pp. 20661–65.

[66]   Bayliss WM. On the local reactions of the arterial wall to changes of internal pressure, *J Physiol*, 1902;28(3): pp. 220–31.

[67]   Bohr DF, Webb RC. Vascular smooth muscle function and its changes in hypertension, *Am J Med*, 1984;77(4A): pp. 3–16.

[68]   Kirber MT, Walsh JV Jr, Singer JJ. Stretch-activated ion channels in smooth muscle: a mechanism for the initiation of stretch-induced contraction, *Pflügers Arch*, 1988;412(4): pp. 339–45.

[69]   Harder DR. Pressure-induced myogenic activation of cat cerebral arteries is dependent on intact endothelium, *Circ Res*, 1987;60(1): pp. 102–07.

[70]   Van Breemen C, Daniel EE. The influence of high potassium depolarization and acetylcholine on calcium exchange in the rat uterus, *J Gen Physiol*, 1966;49(6): pp. 1299–317.

[71]   Somlyo AP, Somlyo AV. Vascular smooth muscle. II. Pharmacology of normal and hypotensive vessels, *Pharmacol Rev*, 1970;22(2): pp. 249–353.

[72] Casteels R, Van Breemen C. Active and passive Ca^{2+} fluxes across cell membranes of the guinea-pig taenia coli, *Pflügers Arch*, 1975;359(3): pp. 197–207.

[73] Raeymaekers L, Wuytack F, Casteels R. Subcellular fractionation of pig stomach smooth muscle. A study of the distribution of the $(Ca^{2++} Mg^{2+})$-ATPase activity in plasmalemma and endoplasmic reticulum, *Biochim Biophys Acta*, 1985;815(3): pp. 441–54.

[74] Rapp JP. Aortic responses to vanadate: independence from (Na,K)-ATPase and comparison of Dahl salt-sensitive and salt-resistant rats, *Hypertension*, 1981;3(3 Pt 2): pp. 1168–72.

[75] Popescu LM, Nutu O, Panoiu C. Oxytocin contracts the human uterus at term by inhibiting the myometrial Ca^{2+}-extrusion pump, *Biosci Rep*, 1985;5(1): pp. 21–28.

[76] Eggermont JA, Vrolix M, Raeymaekers L, Wuytack F, Casteels R. Ca^{2+}-transport ATPases of vascular smooth muscle, *Circ Res*, 1988;62(2): pp. 266–78.

[77] Popescu LM, Ignat P. Calmodulin-dependent Ca^{2+}-pump ATPase of human smooth muscle sarcolemma, *Cell Calcium*, 1983;4(4): pp. 219–35.

[78] Heim R, Iwata T, Zvaritch E, Adamo HP, Rutishauser B, Strehler EE, Guerini D, Carafoli E. Expression, purification, and properties of the plasma membrane Ca^{2+} pump and of its N-terminally truncated 105-kDa fragment, *J Biol Chem*, 1992;267(34): pp. 24476–84.

[79] Kumar R, Haugen JD, Penniston JT. Molecular cloning of a plasma membrane calcium pump from human osteoblasts, *J Bone Miner Res*, 1993;8(4): pp. 505–13.

[80] De Jaegere S, Wuytack F, Eggermont JA, Verboomen H, Casteels R. Molecular cloning and sequencing of the plasma-membrane Ca^{2+} pump of pig smooth muscle, *Biochem J*, 1990;271(3): pp. 655–60.

[81] Grover AK, Kwan CY, Rangachari PK, Daniel EE. Na-Ca exchange in a smooth muscle plasma membrane-enriched fraction, *Am J Physiol*, 1983;244(3): pp. C158–65.

[82] Blaustein MP, Lederer WJ. Sodium/calcium exchange: its physiological implications, *Physiol Rev*, 1999;79(3): pp. 763–854.

[83] Barzilai A, Spanier R, Rahamimoff H. Isolation, purification, and reconstitution of the Na^+ gradient-dependent Ca^{2+} transporter (Na^+–Ca^{2+} exchanger) from brain synaptic plasma membranes, *Proc Natl Acad Sci* USA, 1984;81(20): pp. 6521–25.

[84] Matlib MA, Reeves JP. Solubilization and reconstitution of the sarcolemmal Na^+–Ca^{2+} exchange system of vascular smooth muscle, *Biochim Biophys Acta*, 1987;904(1): pp. 145–48.

[85] Carafoli E, Crompton M. The regulation of intracellular calcium by mitochondria, *Ann N Y Acad Sci*, 1978;307: pp. 269–84.

[86] Reeves JP, Sutko JL. Sodium–calcium exchange activity generates a current in cardiac membrane vesicles, *Science*, 1980;208(4451): pp. 1461–64.

[87] Reeves JP, Hale CC. The stoichiometry of the cardiac sodium–calcium exchange system, *J Biol Chem*, 1984;259(12): pp. 7733–39.

[88] Mulvany MJ, Aalkjaer C, Petersen TT. Intracellular sodium, membrane potential, and contractility of rat mesenteric small arteries, *Circ Res*, 1984;54(6): pp. 740–49.

[89] Ashida T, Blaustein MP. Regulation of cell calcium and contractility in mammalian arterial smooth muscle: the role of sodium–calcium exchange, *J Physiol*, 1987;392: pp. 617–35.

[90] Blaustein MP, Hamlyn JM. Sodium transport inhibition, cell calcium, and hypertension. The natriuretic hormone/Na^+–Ca^{2+} exchange/hypertension hypothesis, *Am J Med*, 1984;77: pp. 45–59.

[91] Inesi G. Mechanism of calcium transport, *Annu Rev Physiol*, 1985;47: pp. 573–601.

[92] Borle AB. Control, modulation, and regulation of cell calcium, *Rev Physiol Biochem Pharmacol*, 1981;90: pp. 13–153.

[93] MacLennan DH, Wong PT. Isolation of a calcium-sequestering protein from sarcoplasmic reticulum, *Proc Natl Acad Sci* USA, 1971;68(6): pp. 1231–35.

[94] Wuytack F, Raeymaekers L, Verbist J, Jones LR, Casteels R. Smooth-muscle endoplasmic reticulum contains a cardiac-like form of calsequestrin, *Biochim Biophys Acta*, 1987;899(2): pp. 151–58.

[95] Waisman DM, Gimble JM, Goodman DB, Rasmussen H. Studies of the Ca^{2+} transport mechanism of human erythrocyte inside-out plasma membrane vesicles. I. Regulation of the Ca^{2+} pump by calmodulin, *J Biol Chem*, 1981;256(1): pp. 409–14.

[96] Puskin JS, Gunter TE, Gunter KK, Russell PR. Evidence for more than one Ca^{2+} transport mechanism in mitochondria, *Biochemistry*, 1976;15(17): pp. 3834–42.

[97] Rasmussen H, Barrett PQ. Calcium messenger system: an integrated view, *Physiol Rev*, 1984;64(3): pp. 938–84.

[98] Carafoli E. Intracellular calcium homeostasis, *Annu Rev Biochem*, 1987;56: pp. 395–433.

[99] Mitchell P. Coupling of phosphorylation to electron and hydrogen transfer by a chemiosmotic type of mechanism, *Nature*, 1961;191: pp. 144–48.

[100] Yamamoto H, van Breemen C. Ca^{2+} compartments in saponin-skinned cultured vascular smooth muscle cells, *J Gen Physiol*, 1986;87(3): pp. 369–89.

[101] Dubyak GR, Scarpa A. Sarcoplasmic Ca^{2+} transients during the contractile cycle of single barnacle muscle fibres: measurements with arsenazo III-injected fibres, *J Muscle Res Cell Motil*, 1982;3(1): pp. 87–112.

[102] Ashley CC. Calcium ion regulation in barnacle muscle fibers and its relation to force development, *Ann N Y Acad Sci*, 1978;307: pp. 308–29.

[103] Blinks JR, Wier WG, Hess P, Prendergast FG. Measurement of Ca^{2+} concentrations in living cells, *Prog Biophys Mol Biol*, 1982;40(1–2): pp. 1–114.

[104] Gasser R, Frey M, Fleckenstein-Grün G. Free calcium in rat papillary muscle at contraction assessed with Ca-selective microelectrodes, *Angiology*, 1989;40(8): pp. 736–42.

[105] Morgan JP, Morgan KG. Stimulus-specific patterns of intracellular calcium levels in smooth muscle of ferret portal vein, *J Physiol*, 1984;351: pp. 155–67.

[106] Tsien RY. Intracellular measurements of ion activities, *Annu Rev Biophys Bioeng*, 1983;12: pp. 91–116.

[107] Grynkiewicz G, Poenie M, Tsien RY. A new generation of Ca^{2+} indicators with greatly improved fluorescence properties, *J Biol Chem*, 1985;260(6): pp. 3440–50.

[108] Kobayashi S, Kanaide H, Nakamura M. Cytosolic-free calcium transients in cultured vascular smooth muscle cells: microfluorometric measurements, *Science*, 1985;229(4713): pp. 553–56.

[109] Himpens B, Casteels R. Measurement by Quin2 of changes of the intracellular calcium concentration in strips of the rabbit ear artery and of the guinea-pig ileum, *Pflügers Arch*, 1987;408(1): pp. 32–37.

[110] Sugiyama T, Yoshizumi M, Takaku F, Urabe H, Tsukakoshi M, Kasuya T, Yazaki Y. The elevation of the cytoplasmic calcium ions in vascular smooth muscle cells in SHR— measurement of the free calcium ions in single living cells by lasermicrofluorospectrometry, *Biochem Biophys Res Commun*, 1986;141(1): pp. 340–45.

[111] Ikebe M, Hartshorne DJ. The role of myosin phosphorylation in the contraction–relaxation cycle of smooth muscle, *Experientia*, 1985;41(8): pp. 1006–10.

[112] Kamm KE, Stull JT. Regulation of smooth muscle contractile elements by second messengers, *Annu Rev Physiol*, 1989;51: pp. 299–313.

[113] Khalil RA, van Breemen C. Intracellular free calcium concentration/force relationship in rabbit inferior vena cava activated by norepinephrine and high K^+, *Pflügers Arch*, 1990;416: pp. 727–34.

[114] DeFeo TT, Morgan KG. Calcium–force relationships as detected with aequorin in two different vascular smooth muscles of the ferret, *J Physiol*, 1985;369: pp. 269–82.

[115] Rembold CM, Murphy RA. Myoplasmic $[Ca^{2+}]$ determines myosin phosphorylation in agonist-stimulated swine arterial smooth muscle, *Circ Res*, 1988;63(3): pp. 593–603.

[116] Himpens B, Matthijs G, Somlyo AV, Butler TM, Somlyo AP. Cytoplasmic free calcium, myosin light chain phosphorylation, and force in phasic and tonic smooth muscle, *J Gen Physiol*, 1988;92(6): pp. 713–29.

[117] Kitazawa T, Gaylinn BD, Denney GH, Somlyo AP. G-protein-mediated Ca^{2+} sensitization of smooth muscle contraction through myosin light chain phosphorylation, *J Biol Chem*, 1991;266(3): pp. 1708–15.

[118] Rembold CM. Modulation of the $[Ca^{2+}]$ sensitivity of myosin phosphorylation in intact swine arterial smooth muscle, *J Physiol*, 1990;429: pp. 77–94.

[119] Suematsu E, Resnick M, Morgan KG. Change of Ca^{2+} requirement for myosin phosphorylation by prostaglandin F2 alpha, *Am J Physiol*, 1991;261(2 Pt 1): pp. C253–58.

[120] Hai CM, Murphy RA. Ca^{2+}, crossbridge phosphorylation, and contraction, *Annu Rev Physiol*, 1989;51: pp. 285–98.

[121] Berridge MJ. Inositol trisphosphate and diacylglycerol as second messengers, *Biochem J*, 1984;220(2): pp. 345–60.

[122] Gong MC, Fuglsang A, Alessi D, Kobayashi S, Cohen P, Somlyo AV, Somlyo AP. Arachidonic acid inhibits myosin light chain phosphatase and sensitizes smooth muscle to calcium, *J Biol Chem*, 1992;267(30): pp. 21492–98.

[123] Inoue M, Kishimoto A, Takai Y, Nishizuka Y. Studies on a cyclic nucleotide-independent protein kinase and its proenzyme in mammalian tissues. II. Proenzyme and its activation by calcium-dependent protease from rat brain, *J Biol Chem*, 1977;252(21): pp. 7610–16.

[124] Nishizuka Y. Intracellular signaling by hydrolysis of phospholipids and activation of PKC, *Science*, 1992; 258: pp. 607–14.

[125] Kanashiro CA, Khalil RA. Signal transduction by protein kinase C in mammalian cells, *Clin Exp Pharmacol Physiol*, 1998;25(12): pp. 974–85.

[126] Newton AC. Protein kinase C: structure, function, and regulation, *J Biol Chem*, 1995;270: pp. 28495–98.

[127] House C, Kemp BE. Protein kinase C contains a pseudosubstrate prototope in its regulatory domain, *Science*, 1987;238: pp. 1726–28.

[128] Hartwig JH, Thelen M, Rosen A, Janmey PA, Nairn AC, Aderem A. MARCKS is an actin filament crosslinking protein regulated by protein kinase C and calcium-calmodulin, *Nature*, 1992;356: pp. 618–22.

[129] Barman SA, Zhu S, White RE. Protein kinase C inhibits BKCa channel activity in pulmonary arterial smooth muscle, *Am J Physiol Lung Cell Mol Physiol*, 2004;286: pp. L149–55.

[130] Cogolludo A, Moreno L, Bosca L, Tamargo J, Perez-Vizcaino F. Thromboxane A2-induced inhibition of voltage-gated K^+ channels and pulmonary vasoconstriction: role of protein kinase Czeta, *Circ Res*, 2003;93(7): pp. 656–63.

[131] Aviv A. Cytosolic Ca^{2+}, Na^+/H^+ antiport, protein kinase C trio in essential hypertension, *Am J Hypertens*, 1994;7(2): pp. 205–12.

[132] Woodsome TP, Eto M, Everett A, Brautigan DL, Kitazawa T. Expression of CPI-17 and myosin phosphatase correlates with Ca^{2+} sensitivity of protein kinase C-induced contraction in rabbit smooth muscle, *J Physiol*, 2001;535(Pt 2): pp. 553–64.

[133] Inagaki M, Yokokura H, Itoh T, Kanmura Y, Kuriyama H, Hidaka H. Purified rabbit brain protein kinase C relaxes skinned vascular smooth muscle and phosphorylates myosin light chain, *Arch Biochem Biophys*, 1987;254(1): pp. 136–41.

[134] Khalil RA, Morgan KG. Imaging of protein kinase C distribution and translocation in living vascular smooth muscle cells, *Circ Res*, 1991;69(6): pp. 1626–31.

[135] Chardonnens D, Lang U, Rossier MF, Capponi AM, Vallotton MB. Inhibitory and stimulatory effects of phorbol ester on vasopressin-induced cellular responses in cultured rat aortic smooth muscle cells, *J Biol Chem*, 1990;265(18): pp. 10451–57.

[136] Watanabe M, Hachiya T, Hagiwara M, Hidaka H. Identification of type III protein kinase C in bovine aortic tissue, *Arch Biochem Biophys*, 1989;273(1): pp. 165–69.

[137] Khalil RA, Lajoie C, Morgan KG. In situ determination of $[Ca^{2+}]_i$ threshold for translocation of the alpha-protein kinase C isoform, *Am J Physiol*, 1994;266(6 Pt 1): pp. C1544–51.

[138] Haller H, Quass P, Lindschau C, Luft FC, Distler A. Platelet-derived growth factor and angiotensin II induce different spatial distribution of protein kinase C-alpha and -beta in vascular smooth muscle cells, *Hypertension*, 1994;23(6 Pt 2): pp. 848–52.

[139] Singer HA, Schworer CM, Sweeley C, Benscoter H. Activation of protein kinase C isozymes by contractile stimuli in arterial smooth muscle, *Arch Biochem Biophys*, 1992;299(2): pp. 320–29.

[140] Ohanian V, Ohanian J, Shaw L, Scarth S, Parker PJ, Heagerty AM. Identification of protein kinase C isoforms in rat mesenteric small arteries and their possible role in agonist-induced contraction, *Circ Res*, 1996;78(5): pp. 806–12.

[141] Liou YM, Morgan KG. Redistribution of protein kinase C isoforms in association with vascular hypertrophy of rat aorta, *Am J Physiol*, 1994;267: pp. C980–89.

[142] Khalil RA, Lajoie C, Resnick MS, Morgan KG. Ca^{2+}-independent isoforms of protein kinase C differentially translocate in smooth muscle, *Am J Physiol*, 1992;263(3 Pt 1): pp. C714–19.

[143] Khalil RA, Morgan KG. Enzyme translocations during smooth muscle activation. In: Barany M, editor, *Biochemistry of Smooth Muscle Contraction*, New York: pp. Academic Press, 1996. pp. 307–18.

[144] Cogolludo A, Moreno L, Lodi F, Tamargo J, Perez-Vizcaino F. Postnatal maturational shift from PKCzeta and voltage-gated K^+ channels to RhoA/Rho kinase in pulmonary vasoconstriction, *Cardiovasc Res*, 2005;66(1): pp. 84–93.

[145] Thelen M, Rosen A, Nairn AC, Aderem A. Regulation by phosphorylation of reversible association of a myristoylated protein kinase C substrate with the plasma membrane, *Nature*, 1991;351(6324): pp. 320–22.

[146] Draeger A, Wray S, Babiychuk EB. Domain architecture of the smooth-muscle plasma membrane: regulation by annexins, *Biochem J*, 2005;387(Pt 2): pp. 309–14.

[147] Cazaubon SM, Parker PJ. Identification of the phosphorylated region responsible for the permissive activation of protein kinase C, *J Biol Chem*, 1993;268(23): pp. 17559–63.

[148] Ron D, Mochly-Rosen D. Agonists and antagonists of protein kinase C function, derived from its binding proteins, *J Biol Chem*, 1994;269(34): pp. 21395–98.

[149] Horowitz A, Menice CB, Laporte R, Morgan KG. Mechanisms of smooth muscle contraction, *Physiol Rev*, 1996;76(4): pp. 967–1003.

[150] Dallas A, Khalil RA. Ca^{2+} antagonist-insensitive coronary smooth muscle contraction involves activation of s-protein kinase C-dependent pathway, *Am J Physiol Cell Physiol*, 2003; 285(6): pp. C1454–63.

[151] McNair LL, Salamanca DA, Khalil RA. Endothelin-1 promotes Ca^{2+} antagonist-insensitive coronary smooth muscle contraction via activation of s-protein kinase C, *Hypertension*, 2004;43(4): pp. 897–904.

[152] Bazzi MD, Nelseusten GL. Protein kinase C interaction with calcium: a phospholipid-dependent process, *Biochemistry*, 1990;29: pp. 7624–30.

[153] Nishizuka Y. Protein kinase C and lipid signaling for sustained cellular responses, *FASEB J*, 1995;9: pp. 484–96.

[154] Edwards AS, Newton AC. Phosphorylation at conserved carboxyl-terminal hydrophobic motif regulates the catalytic and regulatory domains of protein kinase C, *J Biol Chem*, 1997;272: pp. 18382–90.

[155] Eicholtz T, de Bont DB, Widt J, Liskamp RMJ, Ploegh HL. A myristoylated pseudo substrate peptide, a novel protein kinase C inhibitor, *J Biol Chem*, 1993;268: pp. 1982–86.

[156] Clement S, Tasinato A, Boscoboinik D, Azzi A. The effect of a-tocoferol on the synthesis, phosphorylation and activity of protein kinase C in smooth muscle cells after phorbol 12-myristate 13-acetate, *Eur J Biochem*, 1997;246: pp. 745–49.

[157] Khalil RA, Menice CB, Wang CL, Morgan KG. Phosphotyrosine-dependent targeting of mitogen-activated protein kinase in differentiated contractile vascular cells, *Circ Res*, 1995;76(6): pp. 1101–08.

[158] Somlyo AP, Somlyo AV. Ca^{2+} sensitivity of smooth muscle and nonmuscle myosin II: modulated by G proteins, kinases, and myosin phosphatase, *Physiol Rev*, 2003;83: pp. 1325–58.

[159] Hilgers RH, Webb RC. Molecular aspects of arterial smooth muscle contraction: focus on Rho, *Exp Biol Med* (Maywood), 2005;230(11): pp. 829–35.

[160] Budzyn K, Sobey CG. Vascular rho kinases and their potential therapeutic applications, *Curr Opin Drug Discov Devel*, 2007;10(5): pp. 590–96.

[161] Gong MC, Fujihara H, Somlyo AV, Somlyo AP: Translocation of rhoA associated with Ca^{2+} sensitization of smooth muscle, *J Biol Chem*, 1997;272(16): pp. 10704–09.

[162] Loirand G, Guérin P, Pacaud P. Rho kinases in cardiovascular physiology and pathophysiology, *Circ Res*, 2006;98(3): pp. 322–34.

[163] Leung T, Manser E, Tan L, Lim L. A novel serine/threonine kinase binding the Ras-related RhoA GTPase which translocates the kinase to peripheral membranes, *J Biol Chem*, 1995;270: pp. 29051–54.

[164] Matsui T, Amano M, Yamamoto T, Chihara K, Nakafuku M, Ito M, Nakano T, Okawa K, Iwamatsu A, Kaibuchi K. Rho-associated kinase, a novel serine/threonine kinase, as a putative target for small GTP binding protein Rho, *EMBO J*, 1996;15: pp. 2208–16.

[165] Nakagawa O, Fujisawa K, Ishizaki T, Saito Y, Nakao K, Narumiya S. ROCK-I and ROCK-II, two isoforms of Rho-associated coiled-coil forming protein serine/threonine kinase in mice, *FEBS Lett,* 1996; 392: pp. 189–93.

[166] Leung T, Chen XQ, Manser E, Lim L. The p160 RhoA-binding kinase ROK alpha is a member of a kinase family and is involved in the reorganization of the cytoskeleton, *Mol Cell Biol,* 1996; 16: pp. 5313–27.

[167] Wbberley A, Chen Z, Hu E, Hieble JP, Westfall TD. Expression and functional role of Rho-kinase in rat urinary bladder smooth muscle, *Br J Pharmacol,* 2003;138: pp. 757–66.

[168] Hiroki J, Shimokawa H, Higashi M, Morikawa K, Kandabashi T, Kawamura N, Kubota T, Ichiki T, Amano M, Kaibuchi K, Takeshita A. Inflammatory stimuli upregulate Rho-kinase in human coronary vascular smooth muscle cells, *J Mol Cell Cardiol,* 2004;37: pp. 537–46.

[169] Amano M, Chihara K, Nakamura N, Kaneko T, Matsuura Y, Kaibuchi K: The COOH terminus of rho-kinase negatively regulates rho-kinase activity, *J Biol Chem,* 1999;274(45): pp. 32418–24.

[170] Chen XQ, Tan I, Ng CH, Hall C, Lim L, Leung T. Characterization of RhoA-binding kinase ROKalpha implication of the pleckstrin homology domain in ROKalpha function using region-specific antibodies, *J Biol Chem,* 2002;277(15): pp. 12680–88.

[171] Amano M, Chihara K, Kimura K, Fukata Y, Nakamura N, Matsuura Y, Kaibuchi K. Formation of actin stress fibers and focal adhesions enhanced by Rho-kinase, *Science,* 1997; 275(5304): pp. 1308–11.

[172] Amano M, Fukata Y, Kaibuchi K. Regulation and functions of Rho-associated kinase, *Exp Cell Res,* 2000;261: pp. 44–51.

[173] Doran JD, Liu X, Taslimi P, Saadat A, Fox T. New insights into the structure–function relationships of Rho-associated kinase: a thermodynamic and hydrodynamic study of the dimer-to-monomer transition and its kinetic implications, *Biochem J,* 2004;384: pp. 255–62.

[174] Feng J, Ito M, Kureishi Y, Ichikawa K, Amano M, Isaka N, Okawa K, Iwamatsu A, Kaibuchi K, Hartshorne DJ, Nakano T. Rho-associated kinase of chicken gizzard smooth muscle, *J Biol Chem,* 1999;274: pp. 3744–52.

[175] Shirao S, Kashiwagi S, Sato M, Miwa S, Nakao F, Kurokawa T, Todoroki N-Ikeda, Mogami K, Mizukami Y, Kuriyama S, Haze K, Suzuki M, Kobayashi S. Sphingosylphosphorylcholine is a novel messenger for Rho-kinase-mediated Ca^{2+} sensitization in the bovine cerebral artery: unimportant role for protein kinase C, *Circ Res,* 2002;91: pp. 112–19.

[176] Riento K, Guasch RM, Garg R, Jin B, Ridley AJ. RhoE binds to ROCK I and inhibits downstream signaling, *Mol Cell Biol,* 2003;23: pp. 4219–29.

[177] Ward Y, Yap SF, Ravichandran V, Matsumura F, Ito M, Spinelli B, Kelly K. The GTP binding proteins Gem and Rad are negative regulators of the Rho–Rho kinase pathway, *J Cell Biol,* 2002;157: pp. 291–302.

[178] Amano M, Ito M, Kimura K, Fukata Y, Chihara K, Nakano T, Matsuura Y, Kaibuchi K. Phosphorylation and activation of myosin by Rho-associated kinase (Rho-kinase), *J Biol Chem*, 1996;271: pp. 20246–49.

[179] Goto H, Kosako H, Tanabe K, Yanagida M, Sakurai M, Amano M, Kaibuchi K, Inagaki M. Phosphorylation of vimentin by Rho-associated kinase at a unique amino-terminal site that is specifically phosphorylated during cytokinesis, *J Biol Chem*, 1998;273: pp. 11728–36.

[180] Matsui T, Maeda M, Doi Y, Yonemura S, Amano M, Kaibuchi K, Tsukita S, Tsukita S. Rho-kinase phosphorylates COOH-terminal threonines of ezrin/radixin/moesin (ERM) proteins and regulates their head-to-tail association, *J Cell Biol*, 1998;140: pp. 647–57.

[181] Fukata Y, Oshiro N, Kinoshita N, Kawano Y, Matsuoka Y, Bennett V, Matsuura Y, Kaibuchi K. Phosphorylation of adducin by Rho-kinase plays a crucial role in cell motility, *J Cell Biol*, 1999;145: pp. 347–61.

[182] Riento K, Ridley AJ. Rocks: multifunctional kinases in cell behavior, *Nat Rev Mol Cell Biol*, 2003;4:446–56.

[183] Mueller BK, Mack H, Teusch N. Rho kinase, a promising drug target for neurological disorders, *Nat Rev Drug Discov*, 2005;4: pp. 387–98.

[184] Kimura K, Ito M, Amano M, Chihara K, Fukata Y, Nakafuku M, Yamamori B, Feng J, Nakano T, Okawa K, Iwamatsu A, Kaibuchi K. Regulation of myosin phosphatase by Rho and Rho-associated kinase (Rho-kinase), *Science*, 1996;273: pp. 245–48.

[185] Kitazawa T, Eto M, Woodsome TP, Brautigan DL. Agonists trigger G protein-mediated activation of the CPI-17 inhibitor phosphoprotein of myosin light chain phosphatase to enhance vascular smooth muscle contractility, *J Biol Chem*, 2000;275: pp. 9897–9900.

[186] Kaneko T, Amano M, Maeda A, Goto H, Takahashi K, Ito M, Kaibuchi K. Identification of calponin as a novel substrate of Rho-kinase, *Biochem Biophys Res Commun*, 2000;273: pp. 110–16.

[187] Vahebi S, Kobayashi T, Warren CM, de Tombe PP, Solaro RJ. Functional effects of rho-kinase-dependent phosphorylation of specific sites on cardiac troponin, *Circ Res*, 2005; 96: pp. 740–47.

[188] Li Z, Dong X, Wang Z, Liu W, Deng N, Ding Y, Tang L, Hla T, Zeng R, Li L, Wu D. Regulation of PTEN by Rho small GTPases, *Nat Cell Biol*, 2005;7: pp. 399–404.

[189] Wolfrum S, Dendorfer A, Rikitake Y, Stalker TJ, Gong Y, Scalia R, Dominiak P, Liao JK. Inhibition of Rho-kinase leads to rapid activation of phosphatidylinositol 3-kinase/protein kinase Akt and cardiovascular protection, *Arterioscler Thromb Vasc Biol*, 2004;24: pp. 1842–47.

[190] Begum N, Sandu OA, Ito M, Lohmann SM, Smolenski A. Active Rho kinase (ROK-alpha) associates with insulin receptor substrate-1 and inhibits insulin signaling in vascular smooth muscle cells, *J Biol Chem*, 2002;277: pp. 6214–22.

[191] Riento K, Totty N, Villalonga P, Garg R, Guasch R, Ridley AJ. RhoE function is regulated by ROCK I-mediated phosphorylation, *EMBO J*, 2005;24: pp. 1170–80.

[192] Shimizu Y, Thumkeo D, Keel J, Ishizaki T, Oshima H, Oshima M, Noda Y, Matsumura F, Taketo MM, Narumiya S. ROCK-I regulates closure of the eyelids and ventral body wall by inducing assembly of actomyosin bundles, *J Cell Biol*, 2005;168: pp. 941–53.

[193] Thumkeo D, Keel J, Ishizaki T, Hirose M, Nonomura K, Oshima H, Oshima M, Taketo MM, Narumiya S. Targeted disruption of the mouse rho-associated kinase 2 gene results intrauterine growth retardation and fetal death, *Mol Cell Biol*, 2003;23: pp. 5043–55.

[194] Uehata M, Ishizaki T, Satoh H, Ono T, Kawahara T, Morishita T, Tamakawa H, Yamagami K, Inui J, Maekawa M, Narumiya S. Calcium sensitization of smooth muscle mediated by a rho-associated protein kinase in hypertension, *Nature*, 1997;389(6654): pp. 990–94.

[195] Chrissobolis S, Sobey CG. Evidence that rho-kinase activity contributes to cerebral vascular tone in vivo and is enhanced during chronic hypertension: Comparison with protein kinase C, *Circ Res*, 2001;88(8): pp. 774–79.

[196] Jin L, Ying Z, Hilgers RH, Yin J, Zhao X, Imig JD, Webb RC. Increased rhoA/rho-kinase signaling mediates spontaneous tone in aorta from angiotensin II-induced hypertensive rats, *J Pharmacol Exp Ther*, 2006;318(1): pp. 288–95.

[197] Ito K, Hirooka Y, Kishi T, Kimura Y, Kaibuchi K, Shimokawa H, Takeshita A. Rho/rho-kinase pathway in the brainstem contributes to hypertension caused by chronic nitric oxide synthase inhibition, *Hypertension*, 2004;43(2): pp. 156–62.

[198] Moriki N, Ito M, Seko T, Kureishi Y, Okamoto R, Nakakuki T, Kongo M, Isaka N, Kaibuchi K, Nakano T. RhoA activation in vascular smooth muscle cells from stroke-prone spontaneously hypertensive rats, *Hypertens Res*, 2004;27(4): pp. 263–70.

[199] Shin HK, Salomone S, Potts EM, Lee SW, Millican E, Noma K, Huang PL, Boas DA, Liao JK, Moskowitz MA, Ayata C. Rho-kinase inhibition acutely augments blood flow in focal cerebral ischemia via endothelial mechanisms, *J Cereb Blood Flow Metab*, 2007;27(5): pp. 998–1009.

[200] Mita S, Kobayashi N, Yoshida K, Nakano S, Matsuoka H. Cardioprotective mechanisms of rho-kinase inhibition associated with eNOS and oxidative stress-LOX-1 pathway in Dahl salt-sensitive hypertensive rats, *J Hypertens*, 2005;23(1): pp. 87–96.

[201] Davies SP, Reddy H, Caivano M, Cohen P. Specificity and mechanism of action of some commonly used protein kinase inhibitors, *Biochem J*, 2000;351(Pt 1): pp. 95–105.

[202] Budzyn K, Paull M, Marley PD, Sobey CG. Segmental differences in the roles of rho-kinase and protein kinase C in mediating vasoconstriction, *J Pharmacol Exp Ther*, 2006; 317(2): pp. 791–96.

[203] Kandabashi T, Shimokawa H, Miyata K, Kunihiro I, Eto Y, Morishige K, Matsumoto Y,

Obara K, Nakayama K, Takahashi S, Takeshita A. Evidence for protein kinase C-mediated activation of rho-kinase in a porcine model of coronary artery spasm, *Arterioscler Thromb Vasc Biol*, 2003;23(12): pp. 2209–14.

[204] Noma K, Goto C, Nishioka K, Jitsuiki D, Umemura T, Ueda K, Kimura M, Nakagawa K, Oshima T, Chayama K, Yoshizumi M, Liao JK, Higashi Y. Roles of rho-associated kinase and oxidative stress in the pathogenesis of aortic stiffness, *J Am Coll Cardiol*, 2007;49(6): pp. 698–705.

[205] Nohria A, Grunert ME, Rikitake Y, Noma K, Prsic A, Ganz P, Liao JK, Creager MA. Rho kinase inhibition improves endothelial function in human subjects with coronary artery disease, *Circ Res*, 2006;99(12): pp. 1426–32.

[206] Kishi T, Hirooka Y, Masumoto A, Ito K, Kimura Y, Inokuchi K, Tagawa T, Shimokawa H, Takeshita A, Sunagawa K. Rho-kinase inhibitor improves increased vascular resistance and impaired vasodilation of the forearm in patients with heart failure, *Circulation*, 2005;111(21): pp. 2741–47.

[207] Jacobs M, Hayakawa K, Swenson L, Bellon S, Fleming M, Taslimi P, Doran J. The structure of dimeric ROCKI reveals the mechanism for ligand selectivity, *J Biol Chem*, 2006;281(1): pp. 260–68.

[208] Sugiyama T, Yoshizumi M, Takaku F, Urabe H, Tsukakoshi M, Kasuya T, Yazaki Y. The elevation of the cytoplasmic calcium ions in vascular smooth muscle cells in SHR—measurement of the free calcium ions in single living cells by lasermicrofluorospectrometry, *Biochem Biophys Res Commun*, 1986;141(1): pp. 340–45.

[209] Crews JK, Murphy JG, Khalil RA. Gender differences in Ca^{2+} entry mechanisms of vasoconstriction in Wistar–Kyoto and spontaneously hypertensive rats, *Hypertension*, 1999;34(4 Pt 2): pp. 931–36.

[210] Murphy JG, Herrington JN, Granger JP, Khalil RA. Enhanced $[Ca^{2+}]_i$ in renal arterial smooth muscle cells of pregnant rats with reduced uterine perfusion pressure, *Am J Physiol Heart Circ Physiol*, 2003;284(1): pp. H393–403.

[211] Matsui T, Takuwa Y, Johshita H, Yamashita K, Asano T. Possible role of protein kinase C-dependent smooth muscle contraction in the pathogenesis of chronic cerebral vasospasm, *J Cereb Blood Flow Metab*, 1991;11(1): pp. 143–49.

[212] Ito A, Shimokawa H, Nakaike R, Fukai T, Sakata M, Takayanagi T, Egashira K, Takeshita A. Role of protein kinase C-mediated pathway in the pathogenesis of coronary artery spasm in a swine model, *Circulation*, 1994;90(5): pp. 2425–31.

[213] Takagi Y, Hirata Y, Takata S, Yoshimi H, Fukuda Y, Fujita T, Hidaka H. Effects of protein kinase inhibitors on growth factor-stimulated DNA synthesis in cultured rat vascular smooth muscle cells, *Atherosclerosis*, 1988;74(3): pp. 227–30.

[214] Bønaa KH, Bjerve KS, Straume B, Gram IT, Thelle D. Effect of eicosapentaenoic and docosahexaenoic acids on blood pressure in hypertension. A population-based intervention trial from the Tromsø study, *N Engl J Med*, 1990;322(12): pp. 795–801.

[215] Chin JP, Gust AP, Nestel PJ, Dart AM. Marine oils dose-dependently inhibit vasoconstriction of forearm resistance vessels in humans, *Hypertension*, 1993;21(1): pp. 22–28.

[216] Hui R, Robillard M, Falardeau P. Inhibition of vasopressin-induced formation of diradylglycerols in vascular smooth muscle cells by incorporation of eicosapentaenoic acid in membrane phospholipids, *J Hypertens*, 1992;10(10): pp. 1145–53.

[217] Seko T, Ito M, Kureishi Y, Okamoto R, Moriki N, Onishi K, Isaka N, Hartshorne DJ, Nakano T. Activation of RhoA and inhibition of myosin phosphatase as important components in hypertension in vascular smooth muscle, *Circ Res*, 2003;92: pp. 411–18.

[218] Mukai Y, Shimokawa H, Matoba T, Kandabashi T, Satoh S, Hiroki J, Kaibuchi K, Takeshita A. Involvement of Rho-kinase in hypertensive vascular disease: a novel therapeutic target in hypertension, *FASEB J*, 2001;15: pp. 1062–64.

[219] Kataoka C, Egashira K, Inoue S, Takemoto M, Ni W, Koyanagi M, Kitamoto S, Usui M, Kaibuchi K, Shimokawa H, Takeshita A. Important role of Rho-kinase in the pathogenesis of cardiovascular inflammation and remodeling induced by long-term blockade of nitric oxide synthesis in rats, *Hypertension*, 2002;39: pp. 245–50.

[220] Higashi M, Shimokawa H, Hattori T, Hiroki J, Mukai Y, Morikawa K, Ichiki T, Takahashi S, Takeshita A. Long-term inhibition of Rho-kinase suppresses angiotensin II-induced cardiovascular hypertrophy in rats in vivo: effect on endothelial NAD(P)H oxidase system, *Circ Res*, 2003;93: pp. 767–75.

[221] Funakoshi Y, Ichiki T, Shimokawa H, Egashira K, Takeda K, Kaibuchi K, Takeya M, Yoshimura T, Takeshita A. Rho-kinase mediates angiotensin II-induced monocyte chemoattractant protein-1 expression in rat vascular smooth muscle cells, *Hypertension*, 2001;38: pp. 100–04.

[222] Takeda K, Ichiki T, Tokunou T, Iino N, Fujii S, Kitabatake A, Shimokawa H, Takeshita A. Critical role of Rho-kinase and MEK/ERK pathways for angiotensin II-induced plasminogen activator inhibitor type-1 gene expression, *Arterioscler Thromb Vasc Biol*, 2001;21: pp. 868–73.

[223] Hishikawa K, Nakaki T, Marumo T, Hayashi M, Suzuki H, Kato R, Saruta T. Pressure promotes DNA synthesis in rat cultured vascular smooth muscle cells, *J Clin Invest*, 1994;93: pp. 1975–80.

[224] Numaguchi K, Eguchi S, Yamakawa T, Motley ED, Inagami T. Mechanotransduction of rat aortic vascular smooth muscle cells requires RhoA and intact actin filaments, *Circ Res*, 1999;85: pp. 5–11.

[225] Zeidan A, Nordstrom I, Albinsson S, Malmqvist U, Sward K, Hellstrand P. Stretch-induced contractile differentiation of vascular smooth muscle: sensitivity to actin polymerization inhibitors, *Am J Physiol Cell Physiol*, 2003;284: pp. C1387–96.

[226] Mandegar M, Fung YC, Huang W, Remillard CV, Rubin LJ, Yuan JX. Cellular and molecular mechanisms of pulmonary vascular remodeling: role in the development of pulmonary hypertension, *Microvasc Res*, 2004;68: pp. 75–103.

[227] Takemoto M, Sun J, Hiroki J, Shimokawa H, Liao JK. Rho-kinase mediates hypoxia-induced downregulation of endothelial nitric oxide synthase, *Circulation*, 2002;106: pp. 57–62.

[228] Guilluy C, Sauzeau V, Rolli-Derkinderen M, Guerin P, Sagan C, Pacaud P, Loirand G. Inhibition of RhoA/Rho kinase pathway is involved in the beneficial effect of sildenafil on pulmonary hypertension, *Br J Pharmacol*, 2005;146: pp. 1010–18.

[229] Nagaoka T, Fagan KA, Gebb SA, Morris KG, Suzuki T, Shimokawa H, McMurtry IF, Oka M. Inhaled Rho kinase inhibitors are potent and selective vasodilators in rat pulmonary hypertension, *Am J Respir Crit Care Med*, 2005;171: pp. 494–99.

[230] Fagan KA, Oka M, Bauer NR, Gebb SA, Ivy DD, Morris KG, McMurtry IF. Attenuation of acute hypoxic pulmonary vasoconstriction and hypoxic pulmonary hypertension in mice by inhibition of Rho-kinase, *Am J Physiol Lung Cell Mol Physiol*, 2004;287: pp. L656–64.

[231] Jernigan NL, Walker BR, Resta TC. Chronic hypoxia augments protein kinase G-mediated Ca^{2+} desensitization in pulmonary vascular smooth muscle through inhibition of RhoA/Rho kinase signaling, *Am J Physiol Lung Cell Mol Physiol*, 2004;287: pp. L1220–29.

[232] Nagaoka T, Morio Y, Casanova N, Bauer N, Gebb S, McMurtry I, Oka M. Rho/Rho kinase signaling mediates increased basal pulmonary vascular tone in chronically hypoxic rats, *Am J Physiol Lung Cell Mol Physiol*, 2004;287: pp. L665–72.

[233] Abe K, Shimokawa H, Morikawa K, Uwatoku T, Oi K, Matsumoto Y, Hattori T, Nakashima Y, Kaibuchi K, Sueishi K, Takeshita A. Long-term treatment with a Rho-kinase inhibitor improves monocrotaline-induced fatal pulmonary hypertension in rats, *Circ Res*, 2004;94: pp. 385–93.

Author Biography

Dr. Raouf Khalil is an assistant professor of surgery at Harvard Medical School and Brigham and Women's Hospital in Boston, MA. He earned his medical degree from Cairo University, completing a medicine internship at Kasr El-Eini Hospital and a medical residency at the Ministry of Public Health, both in Cairo. Dr. Khalil received his PhD from the University of Miami School of Medicine and did postdoctoral work at Harvard Medical School and Beth Israel Hospital. Before returning to Harvard Medical School to his current position, Dr. Khalil held other academic and research positions at the University of Mississippi Medical Center and the VA Boston Healthcare System.

The main focus of Dr. Khalil's research in the vascular surgery laboratory is to study the cellular mechanisms of vascular tone under physiological conditions and the changes in these mechanisms in pathological conditions such as coronary artery disease, salt-sensitive hypertension, abdominal aortic aneurysm, varicose veins, and other chronic vascular diseases. His present research projects include investigation of endothelium-dependent mechanisms of vascular relaxation, Ca^{2+}-dependent and Ca^{2+}-independent mechanisms of vascular contraction, role of protein kinases and phosphatases in vascular smooth muscle contraction, mechanisms of gender-specific differences in vascular tone, role of endothelin in salt-sensitive hypertension, and the cellular mechanisms responsible for vascular aneurysm formation, varicose veins, and other inflammatory vascular disorders. Dr. Khalil's research has been funded by grant awards from the National Institutes of Health (NIH), American Heart Association (AHA), and other funding organizations. In addition, he has mentored and trained more than 40 U.S. and international undergraduate, graduate, medical, and postdoctoral trainees. He has also published more than 100 scientific articles, abstracts, and books, and has taught and given presentations both nationally and internationally at seminars and conferences.

Dr. Khalil is a reviewer for many professional journals and serves on the editorial boards of several journals such as *American Journal of Physiology, Biochemical Pharmacology,* and *Circulation Research* and as associate editor of the *Journal of Pharmacology & Experimental Therapeutics* and section editor of the cardiovascular pharmacology section of the *Open Pharmacology Journal.* He is a fellow of the Council for High Blood Pressure Research and is a member of several professional societies, including the American Heart Association Council on Basic Sciences and the American Physiological Society. He served as chair of the Membership Committee of the American Physiological Society and on several NIH and AHA study groups including the NIH Vascular Cell and Molecular Biology Study Section, and Pregnancy and Neonatology Study Section and the AHA Vascular Biology and Hypertension Study Group.